Contents

FASHION WIGS

Joanne Gale

FASHION WIGS:
selling and servicing

HEINEMANN · LONDON

To Jenny
in gratitude
for her patience
and camera wizardry

W H

William Heinemann Ltd
15 Queen St, Mayfair, London W1X 8BE

LONDON MELBOURNE TORONTO
JOHANNESBURG AUCKLAND

First published 1972

434 90640 9

Photoset and printed in Great Britain by
BAS Printers Limited,
Wallop, Hampshire

Introduction—A New Industry is Born

Throughout the centuries, hair wigs and hairpieces have swept in and out of fashion, according to the prevailing social conditions. Until the early 1950s, though, they were all made by hand. About that time, however, came word of experiments in Hong Kong with machine-made wigs. But it was not for another eleven years that mass-produced wigs and hairpieces were launched in any volume on the world market.

Made from coarse Asian hair, refined to the finer texture of Western hair, they were cheap enough for the

1 Stretch-base Asian hair wig.

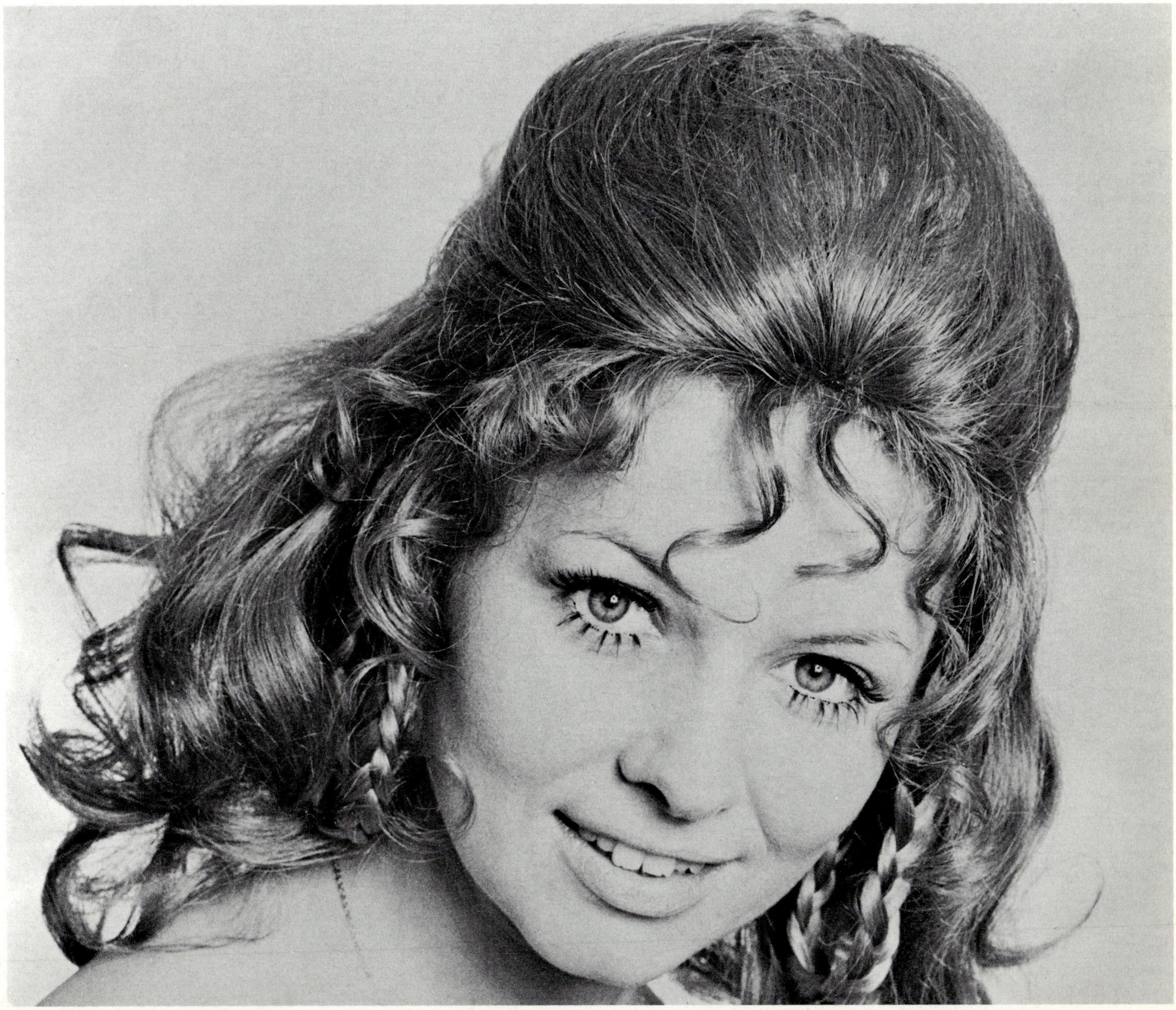

woman in the street and, of course, a novelty. Teenagers went mad about them, followed closely by other age groups. In no time at all they had infiltrated into the fashion scene, even appearing on royal heads. A new industry was born.

An international colour code, originating in France, was worked out, covering a range of 107 hair shades. (This has now been extended to 120 colours.) Wigs and hairpieces, therefore, soon became one of Hong Kong's fastest growing exports—by 1970 employing 24,000 workers. In 1963 British imports of wigs, raw hair, and

2 Teenage design in Asian hair with a stretch base.

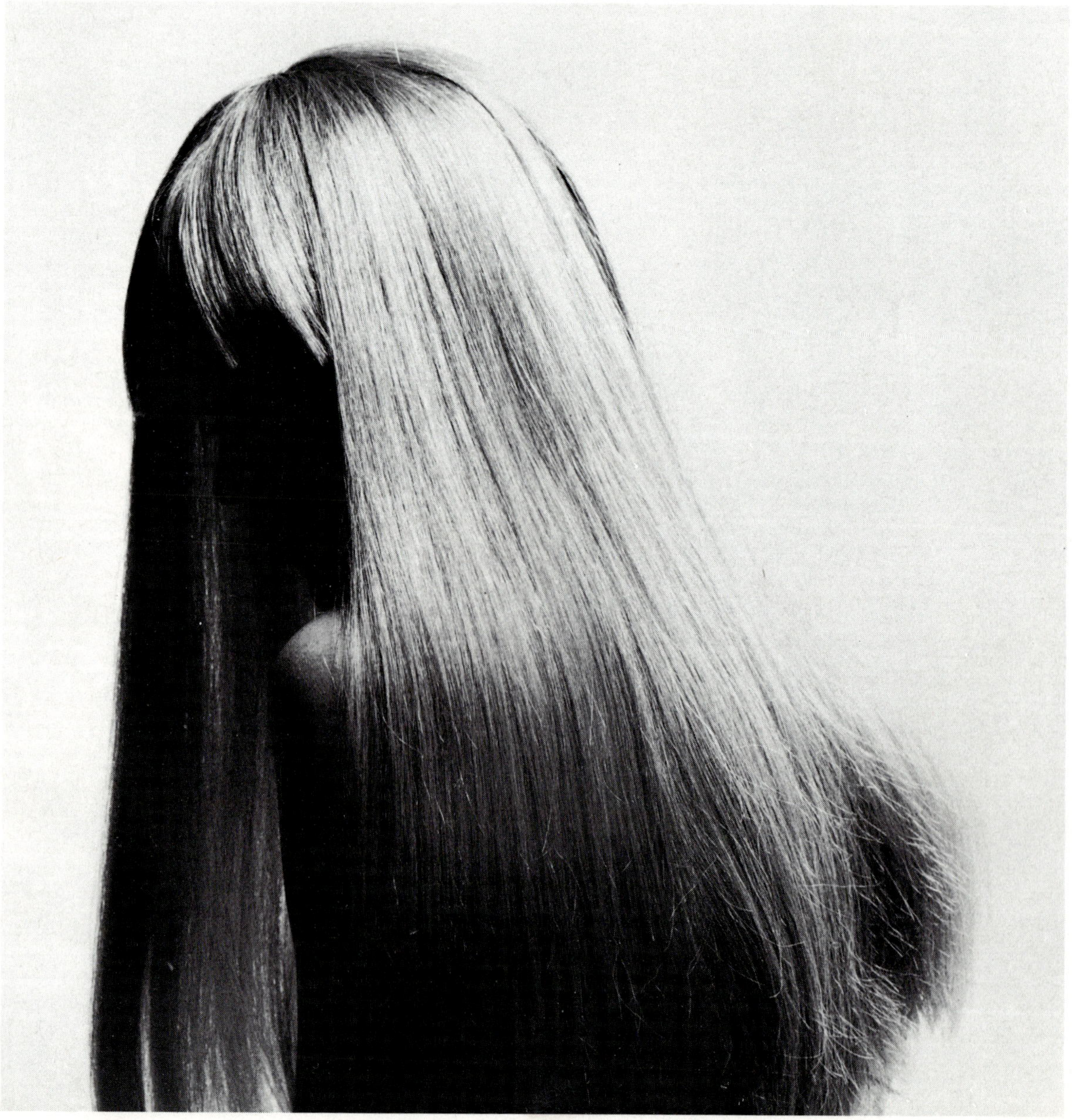

beards, hair pads, curls, switches, etc. from Hong Kong totalled £200,000. By 1966 the figure had risen to £860,000. From there, imports leaped to £2,319,000 the following year, reaching an all-time peak of £4,993,286 in 1968. U.S. imports rose from £3·5 million in 1966 to £9·9 million in 1967, and then jumped by 59 per cent the following year.

This rocketing world demand, already causing a shortage of Asian hair, was given a further boost, early in 1968, by the introduction of wigs with stretch foundations. Up to then, bases had all been one size with somewhat clumsy adjustments at the nape.

3 Hand-made and machine-made bases for hairpieces (*above*) and wigs (*below*): differences in construction.

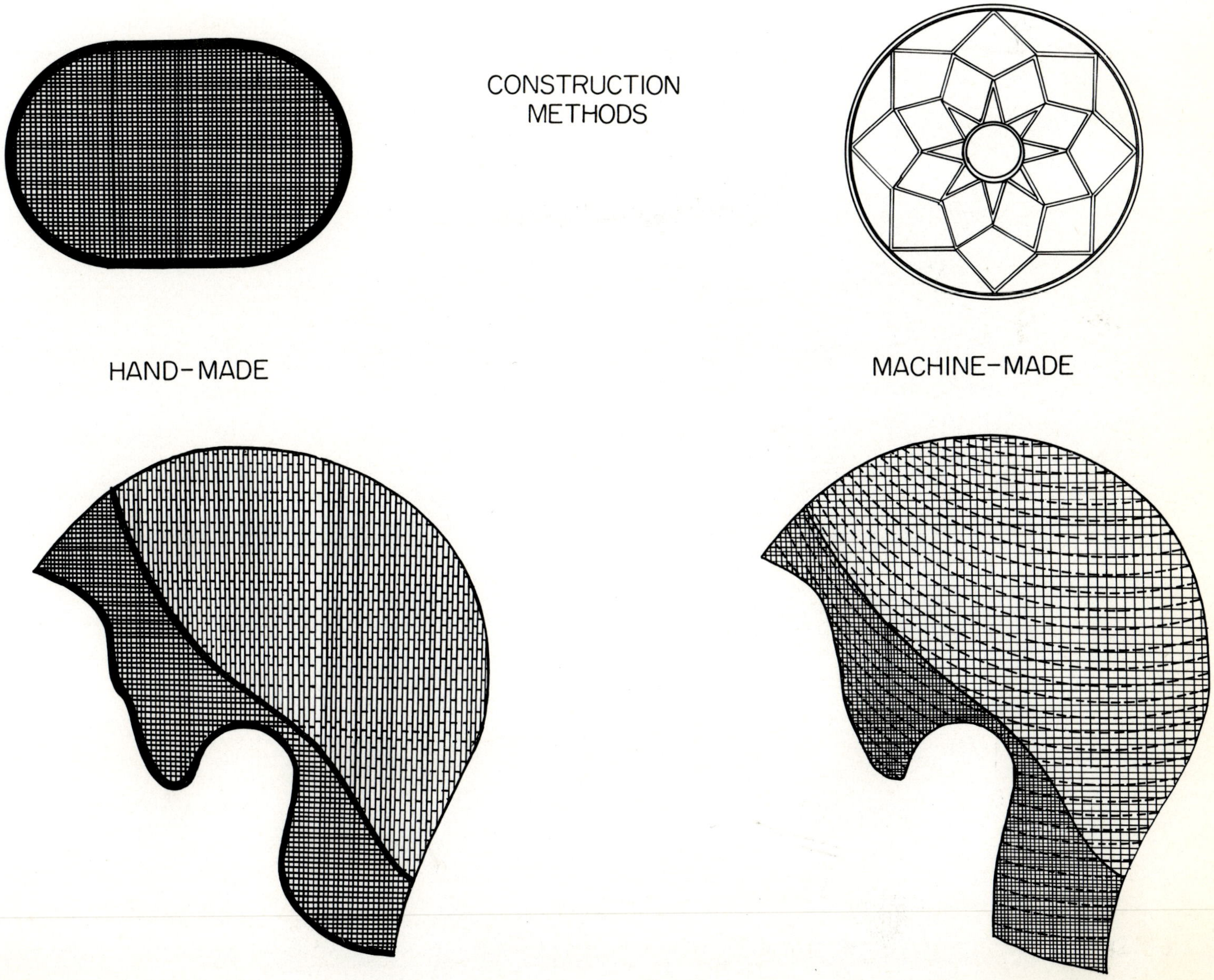

4 Early wig foundations (*left*) and one of today's patterns (*right*)—which are much more comfortable and lie flatter round the hairline.

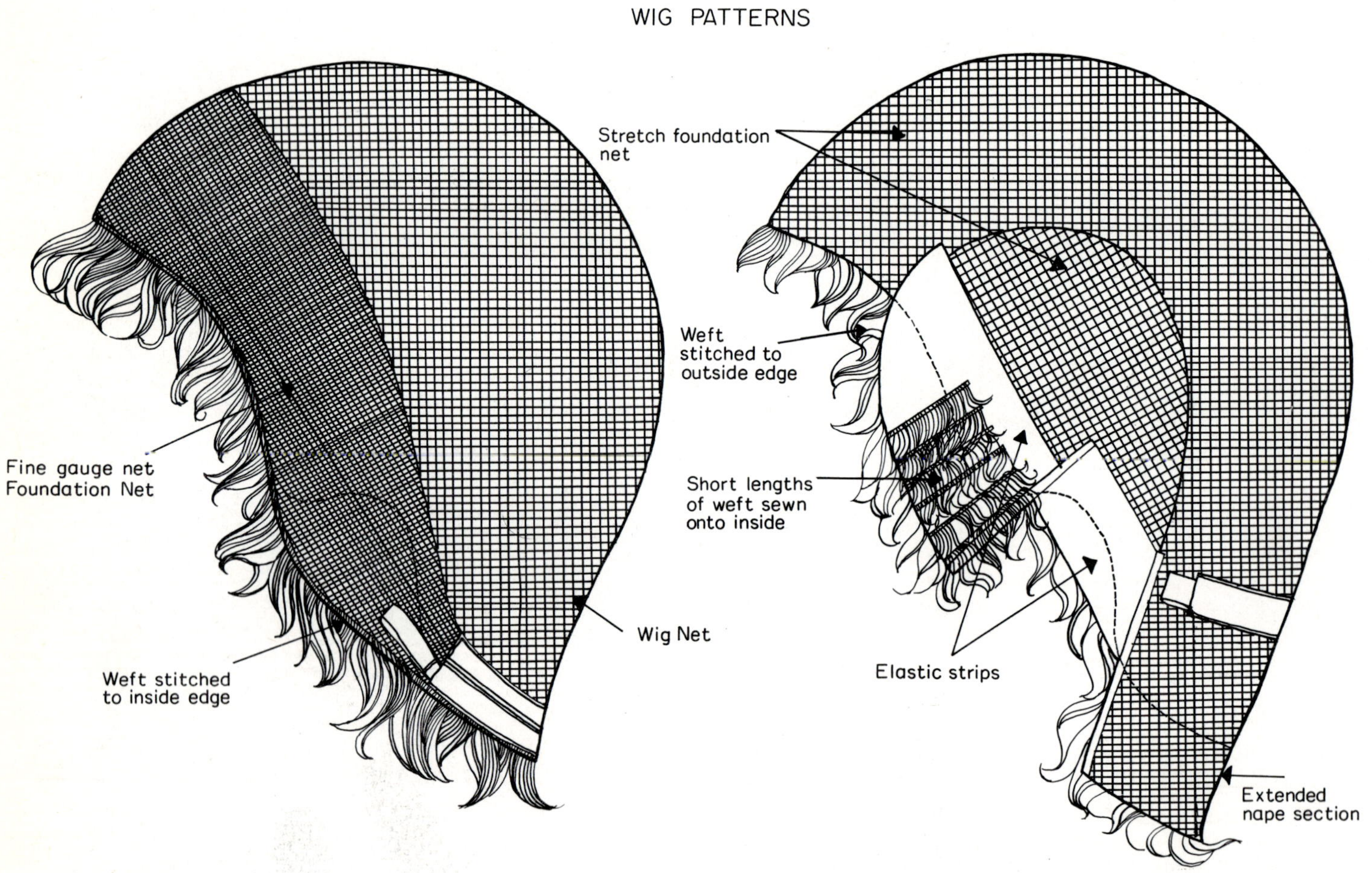

5 (*opposite*) Ready-to-wear wig with a stretch base and mixed modacrylic.

Six months later, synthetic fibre hair appeared on the scene and solved the problem of dwindling Asian hair supplies. Because of its cheapness and washability,

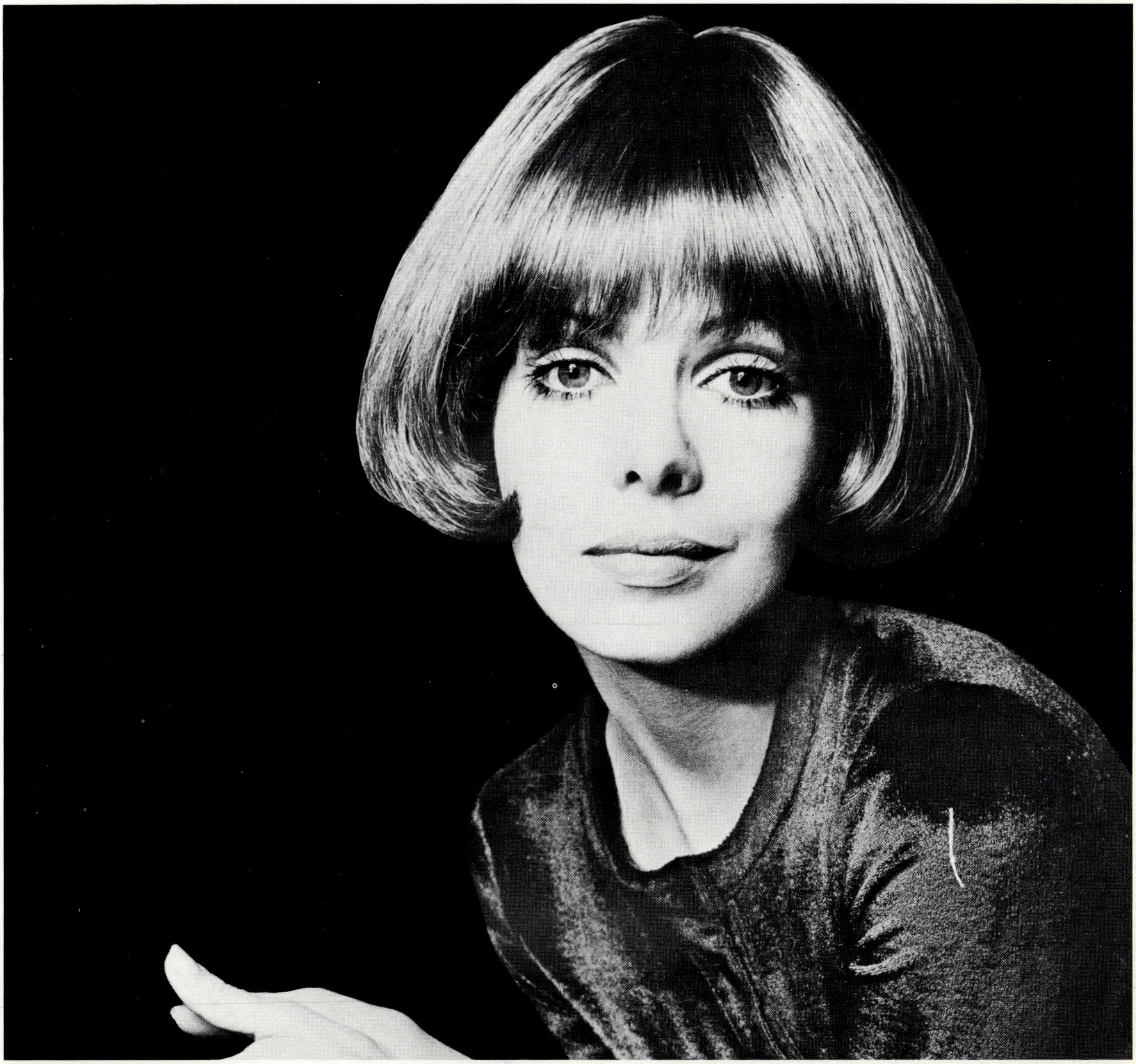

synthetic fibre hair was an overnight success. A 100 per cent growth was the result and, by 1969, between 30 to 40 per cent of total wig production was in fibre. This, by 1970 had reached 70 per cent.

6 Stretch-base, short, ready-to-wear wig in Elura modacrylic.

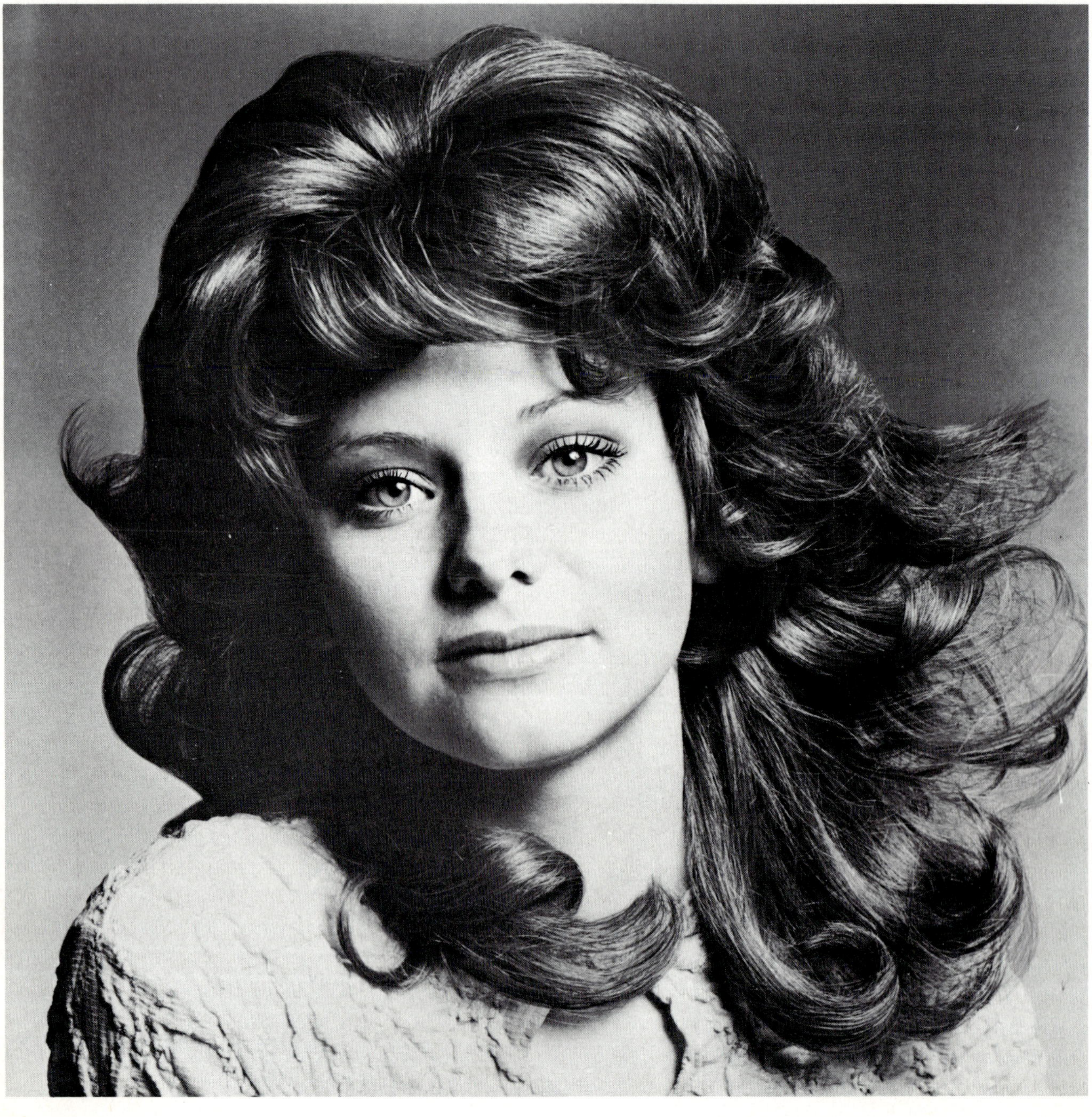

This, then, is the success story of the mass-produced fashion wig. From out of nowhere it has become part of everyday living. Therefore, while hair continues to play a major role in the Total Look of fashion, so there is an expanding market for those involved in selling and servicing added hair.

7 Hairpiece of Asian hair fixed on to the back of the head and styled by a professional.

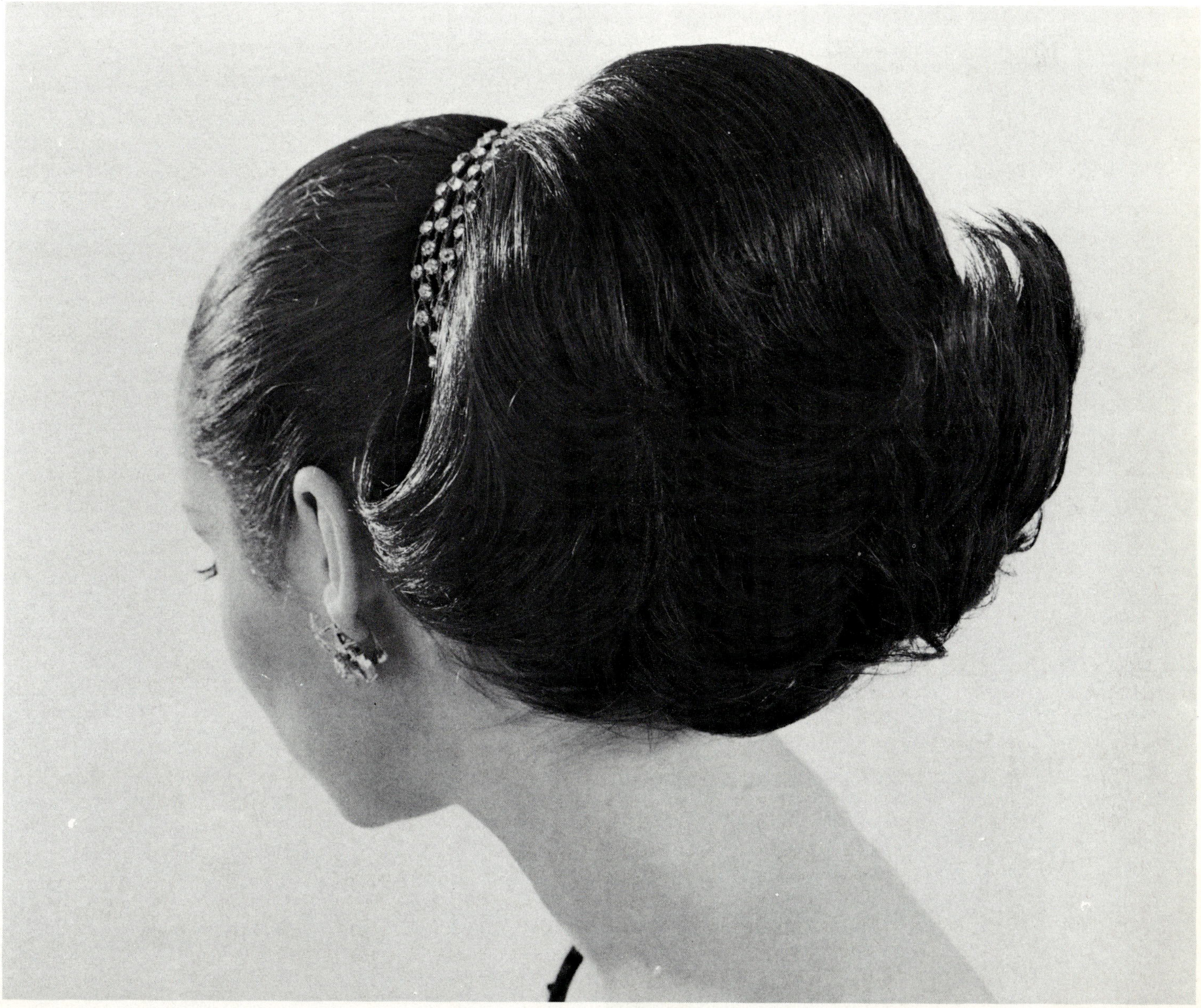

Added Hair—Real and Synthetic

The hair used in fashion wigs is divided into three main categories. First in popularity are the synthetic fibres; second comes Asian hair; and third, because of price, European. Animal hair, too, is also used, but only to a minor degree.

To the non-expert, it all looks very similar. However, there are structural differences as shown by these electron microscope photographs.

European hair

Hair from European sources has the finest texture and is the most expensive in the world. The best comes from Italy and Germany and second quality from France, Spain, Portugal, and mid-Europe. It is usually made up into wigs in its natural state, although some of the lower quality is often curled or re-coloured.

8 European hair—untreated.
Closely resembling natural hair; note the fairly tight overlapping of the cuticle scales. The specks are minute particles of dirt on the strand. The hair is in excellent condition and can be safely bleached, tinted or permed.

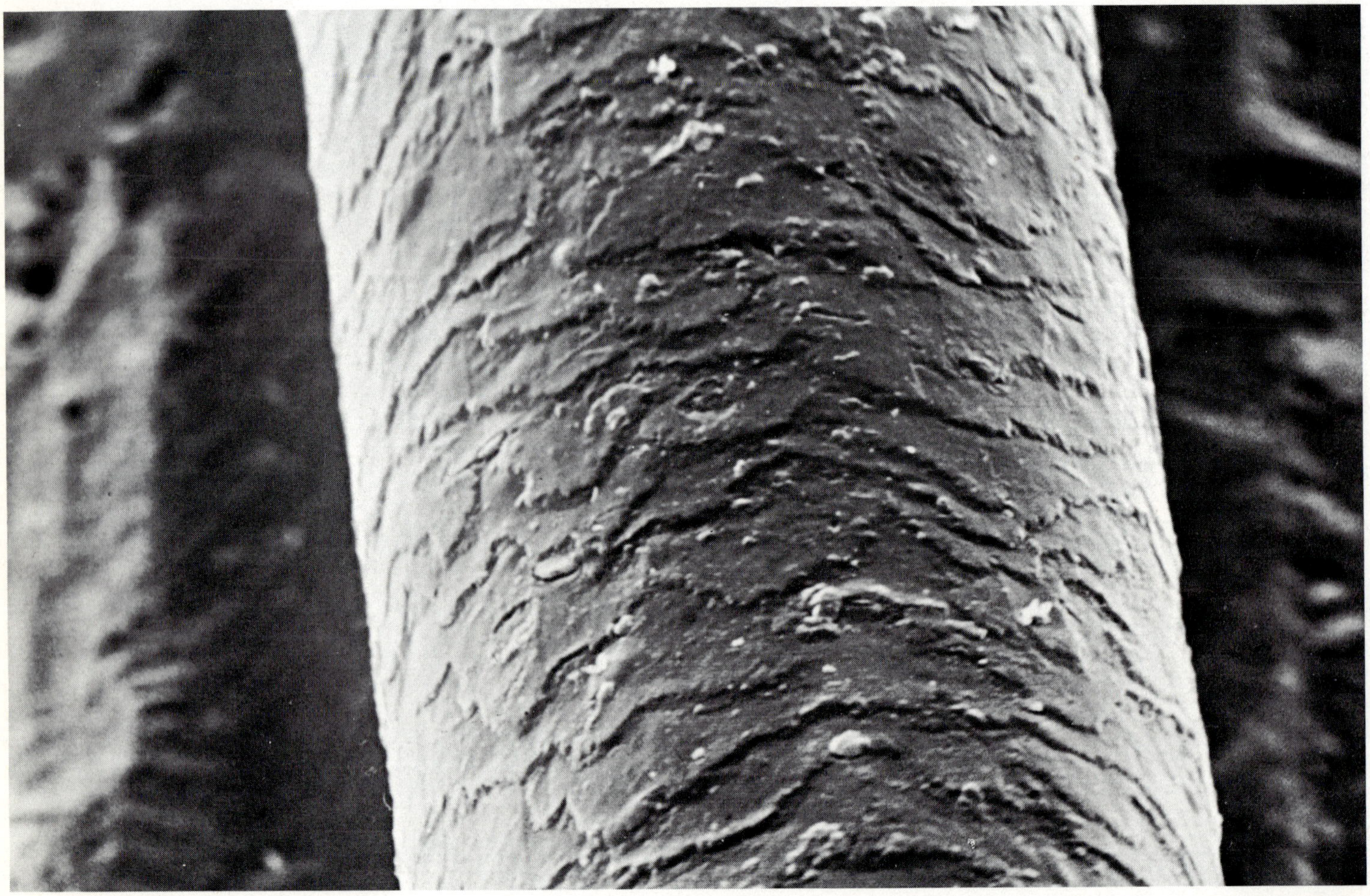

9 European hair—treated.
This hair has been permed which causes scale distortion appearing like ripples across the length of the strand. Dust particles and debris can be seen clinging to it. However, it is in good condition and can be safely tinted or bleached.

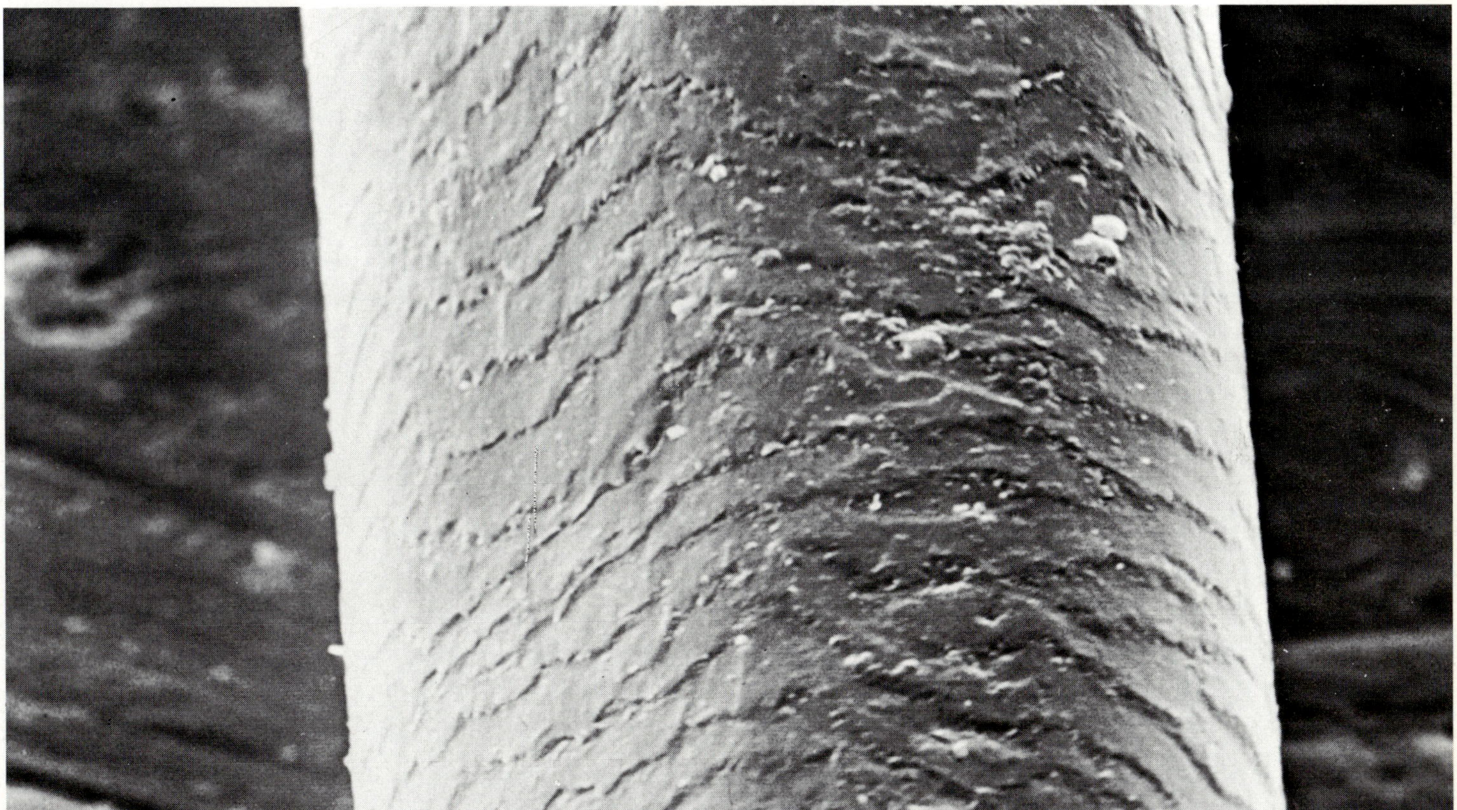

Asian hair

Asian hair is extremely wiry and considerably thicker than Western hair. Either very dark brown or black, it is exported in two forms. One, in its raw state when it is sold for specialized wigmaking, mainly for theatrical or display wigs. Two, made up into fashion wigs. The hair is first put through drastic processing to soften and refine it and then bleached and re-dyed to cater for world variations in hair shades.

10 Asian hair—untreated.
Much coarser than Western hair, it has the normal cuticle with horny overlapping scales. This overlap is, as you can see, fairly firm. The other objects are pieces of dirt still clinging to the strand.

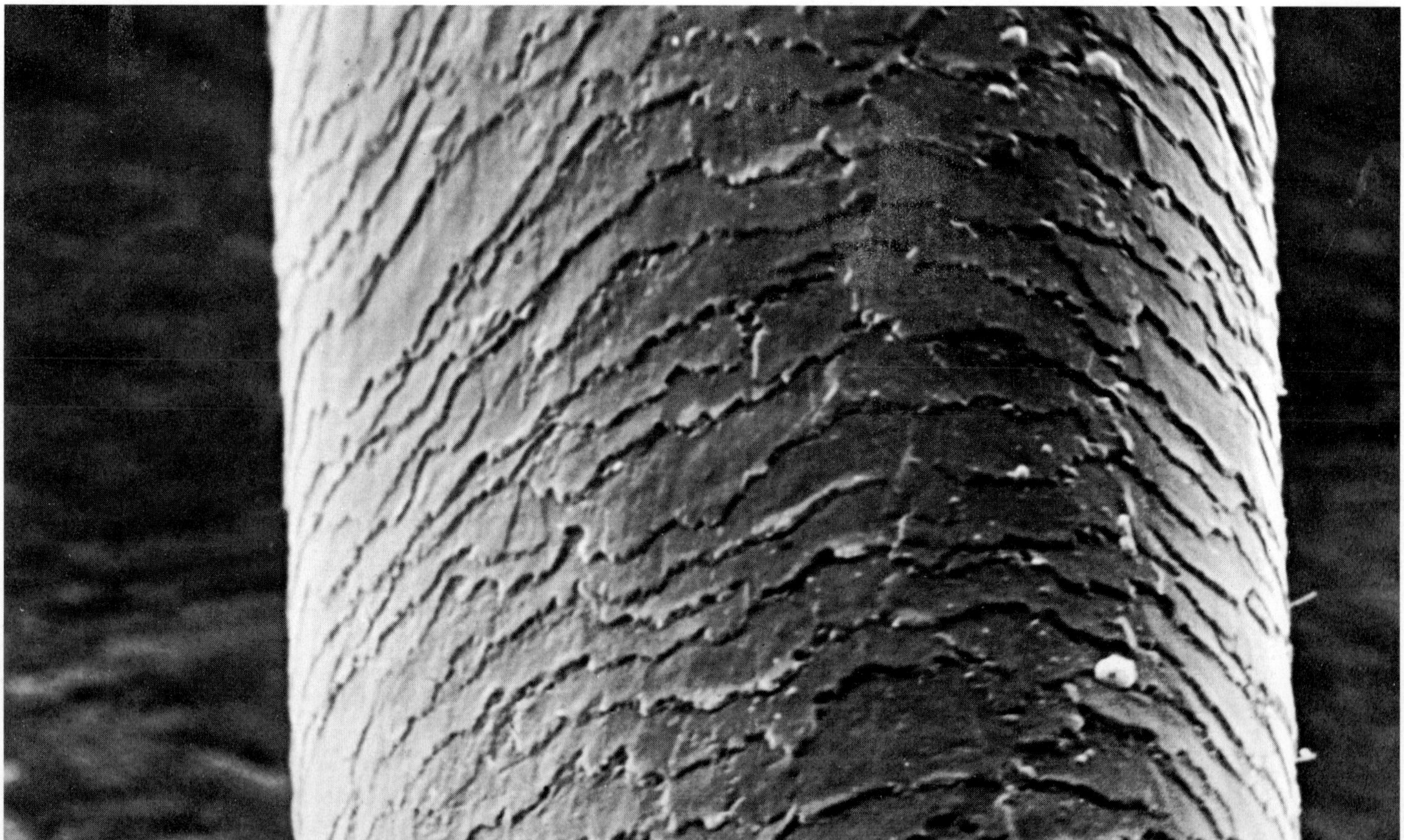

11 Asian hair—treated.

The damage caused to the hair by severe refining processes before making up into wigs is clearly shown. The cuticle scales have been lifted away from the body and, as a result, the hair has become extremely porous. No further hairdressing processing, such as colouring, bleaching or perming, therefore, should be attempted without thorough prior testing.

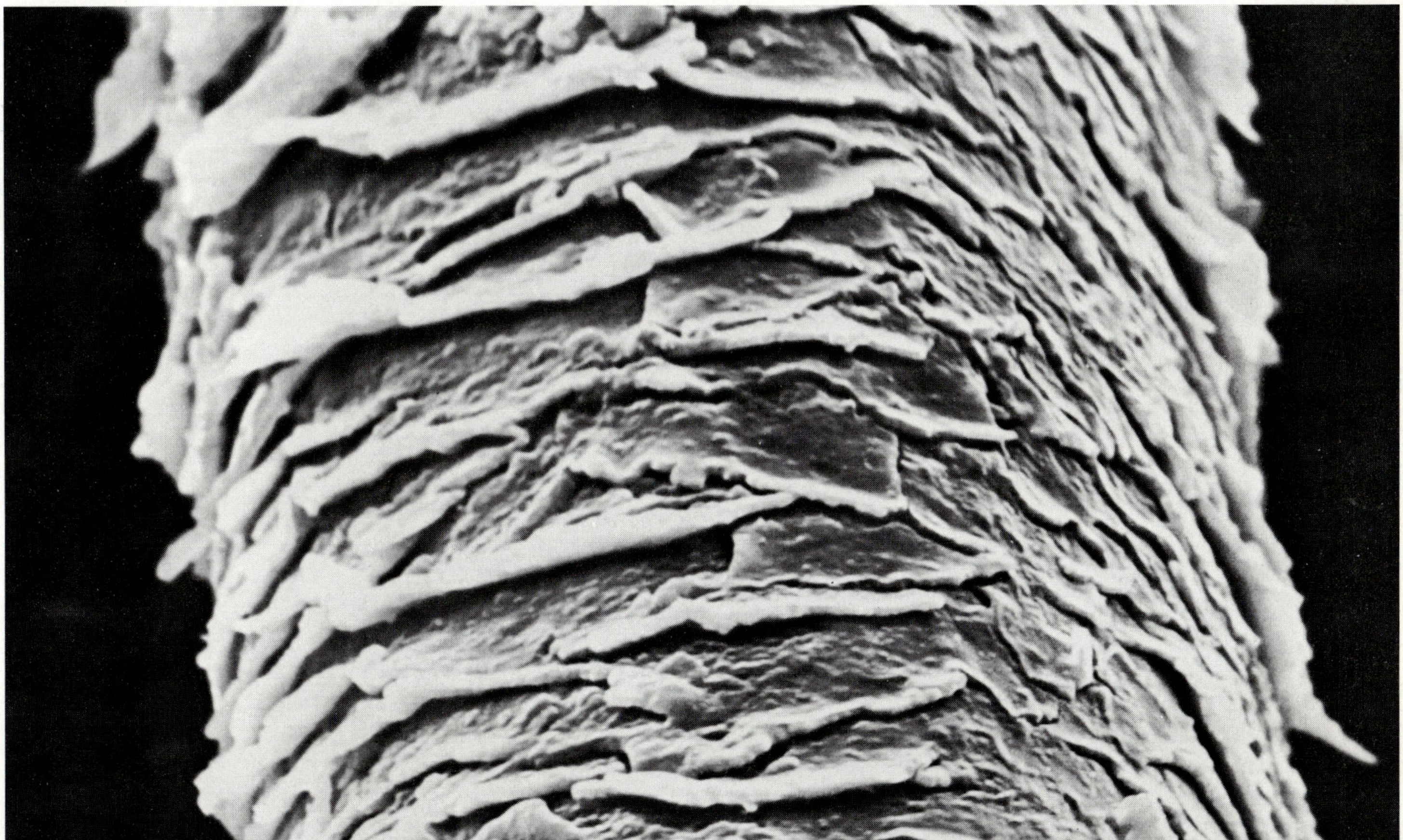

Fibre hair

Progress in research by leading world synthetic fibre manufacturers has resulted in the production of synthetic fibre hair for wigs, closely resembling the look and feel of the hair of humans. This discovery revolutionized the wig market by the introduction of washable wigs.

12 Synthetic fibre hair.
Good synthetic fibre hair is made from acrylic fibre like this in modified forms. Note the absence of cuticle scales showing that its structure differs completely from natural hair. Its external appearance, though, is similar but tinting, bleaching or perming should *never* be attempted.

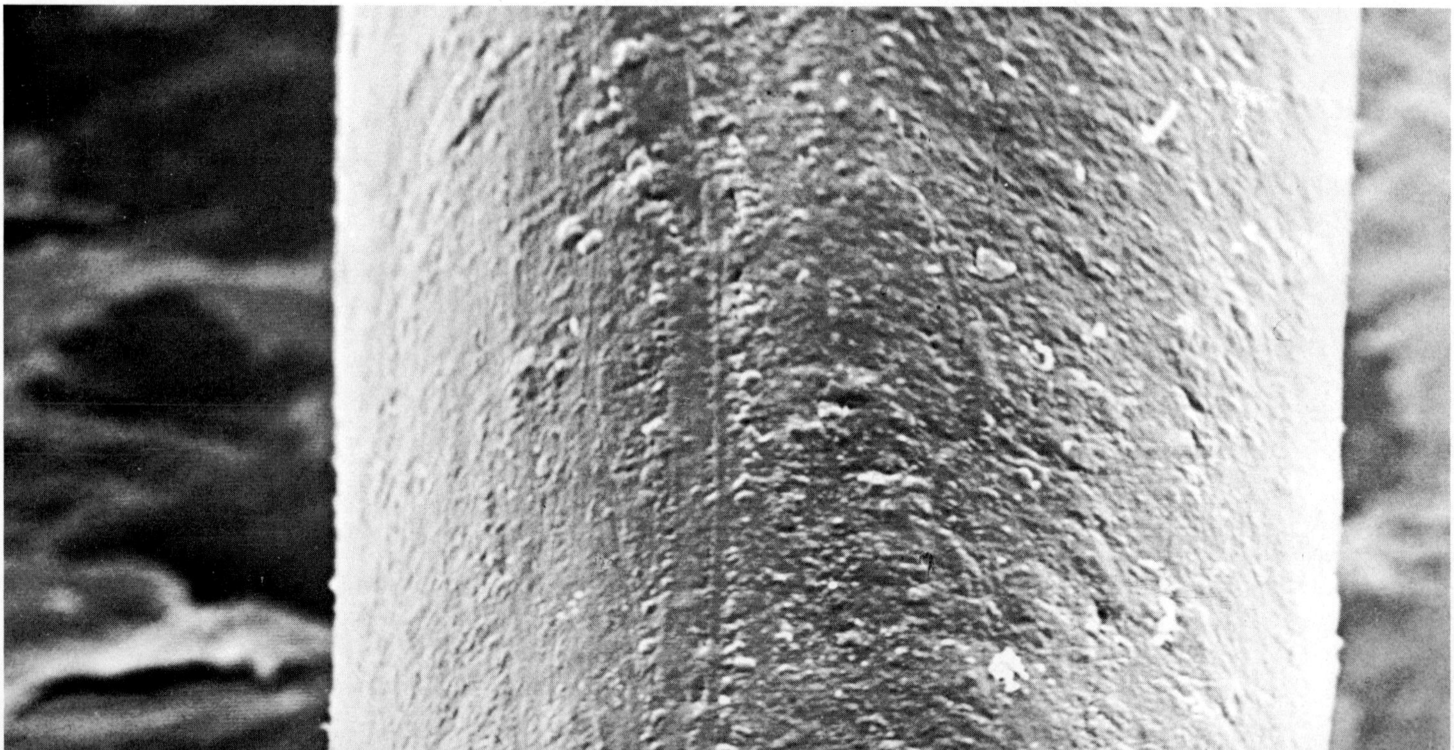

Animal hair

Hair from the yak in its natural state is used for specialist wigmaking. Extremely coarse, it appeared as a blend in early inferior wigs. Today its main use is for theatrical or display wigs and tightly curled, Afro-style, trend wigs.

13 Animal hair.
This strand of hair taken from a yak shows that there is no resemblance between human and animal hair. Nevertheless hair of this type can be tinted or permed, but only by an expert.

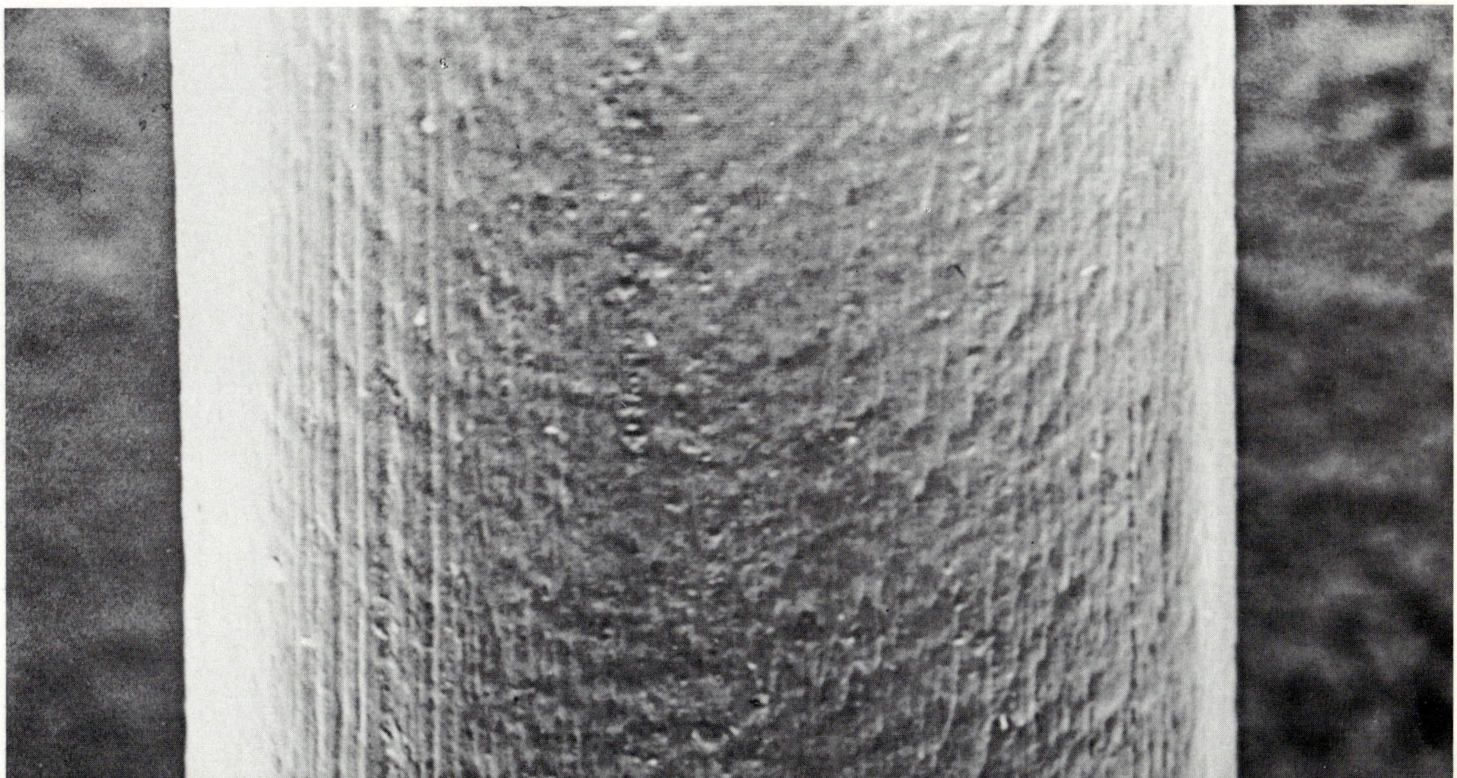

Fibre Hair—Then and Now

The earliest synthetic fibre hair for wigs was made from nylon, nylon blends, and acetates. It looked and felt highly artificial, most of it coarse and flyaway with a very high gloss. Although it was claimed to be washable, severe tangling and crinkling often resulted.

14 Ready-styled wig in Dynel modacrylic fibre.

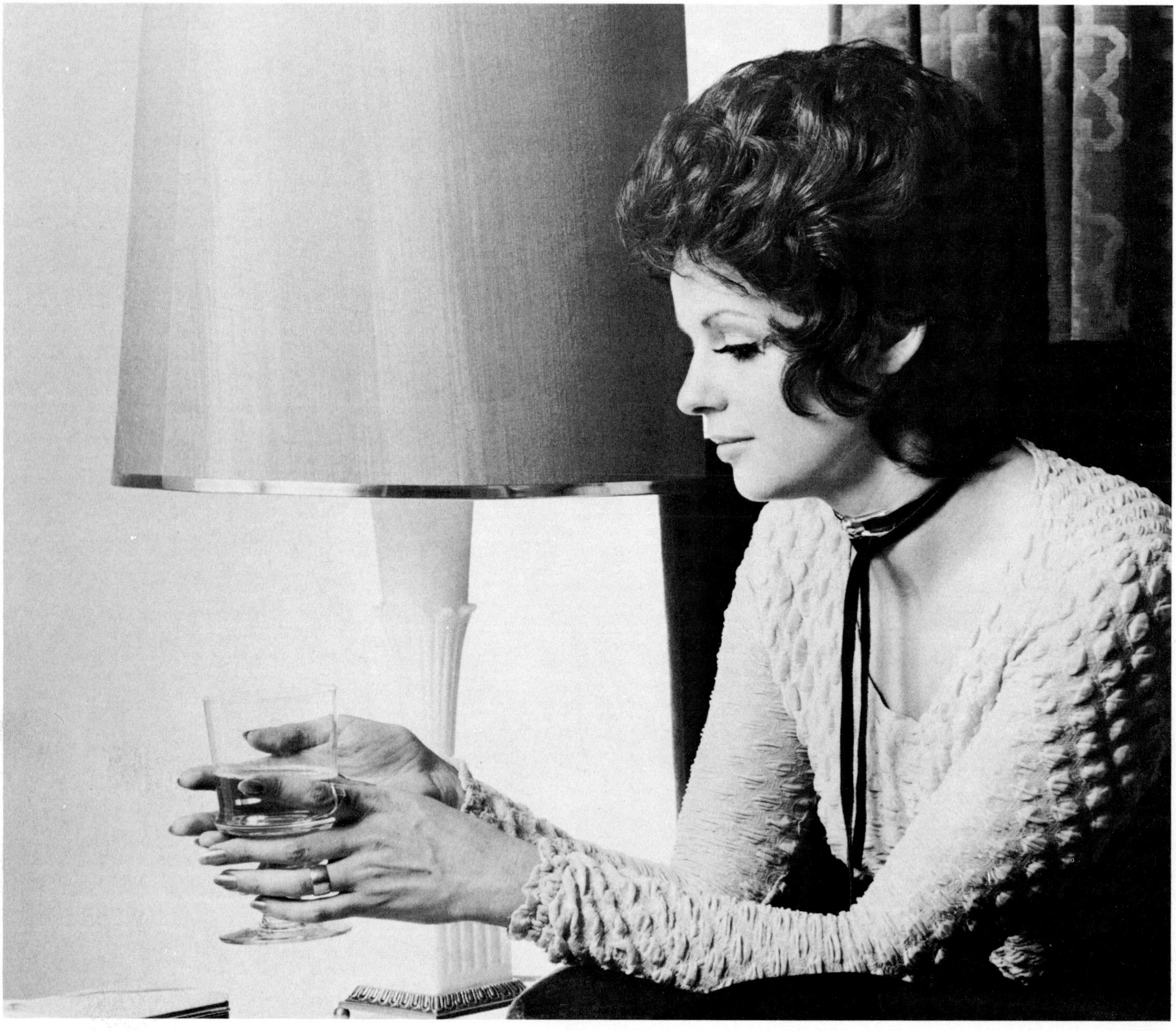

The next hair fibre group to be introduced was the acrylics. They, in the main, were an improvement on the nylons, but earlier ones still left a lot to be desired. Soon afterwards, however, two companies at opposite ends of the world launched first-class modifications, called modacrylics. One was the American Dynel, the other was the Japanese Kanekalon, and each was an overnight success.

These modacrylics looked very natural and washed well, and the movement or modified curl, put in during manufacture, bounced back afterwards. The other big selling point was the price, then much lower than Asian hair. From then on, fibre wig production quickly overtook hair, accounting for about 70 per cent of total wig production by 1970. Other countries introduced fibre hair but Dynel and Kanekalon retained their individual lead.

15 Pull-on wig in Kanekalon modacrylic fibre.

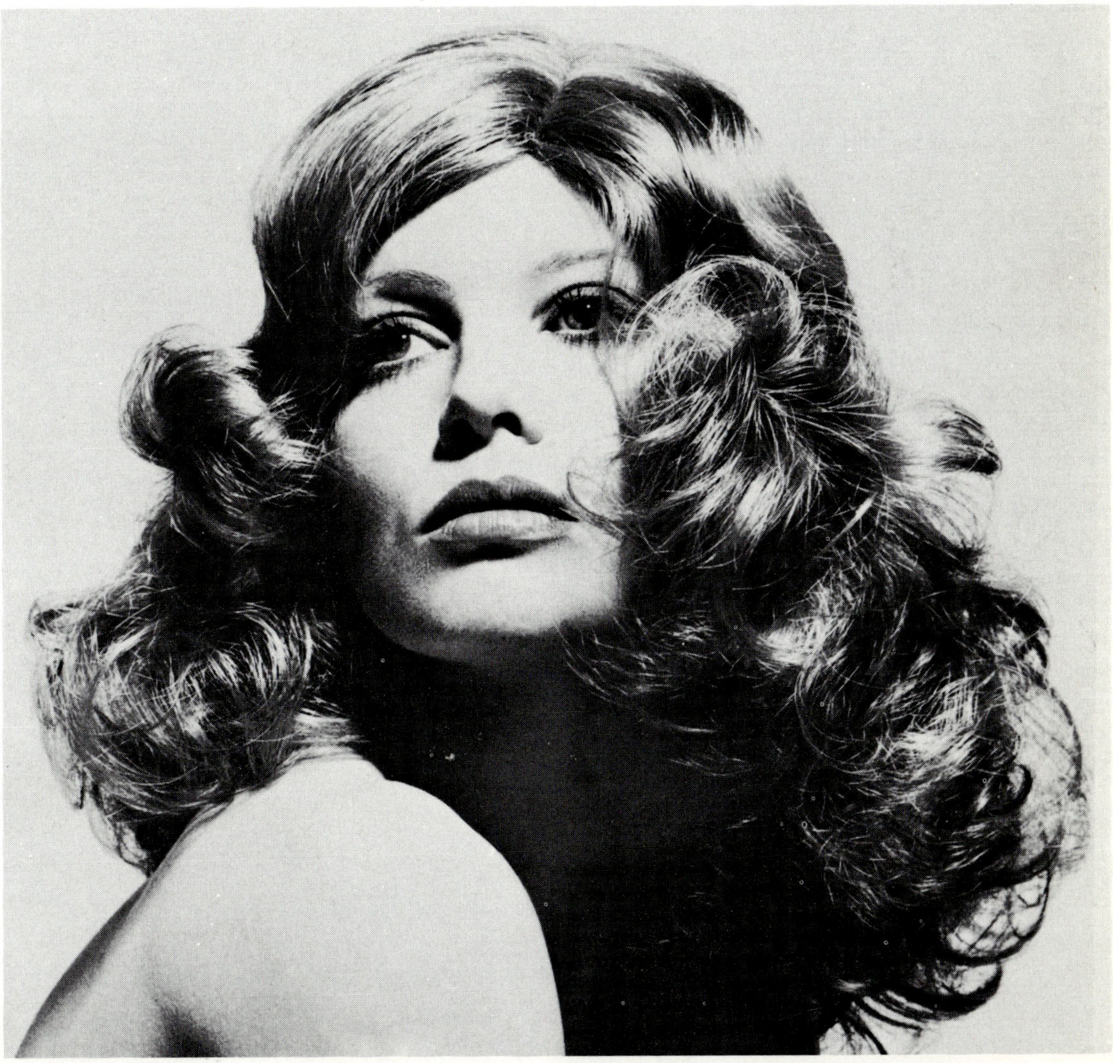

As synthetic hair research progresses, fibre wigs continue to dominate the scene. The launch, in Britain, in 1971 of a second American modacrylic fibre Elura, with cuticle-like surface and ability to withstand more heat, was yet another step towards the goal of perfect hair simulation.

16 Ready-to-wear design in Elura modacrylic fibre.

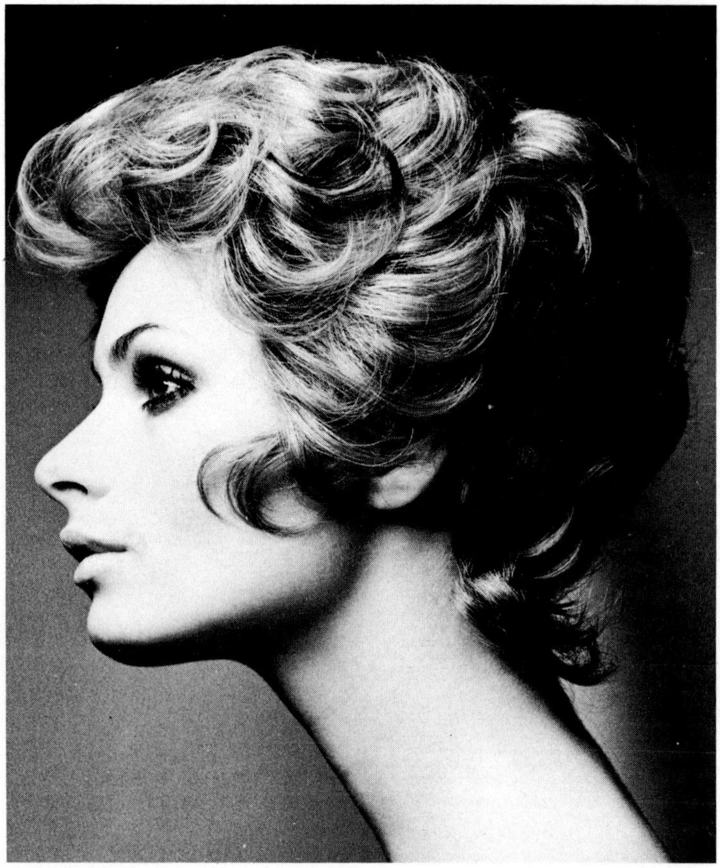

After-care rules

Although modacrylic wigs are washable, easy to care for,* and usually have instructions attached, never assume that these will be read! Each time a wig of this type is sold, the following basic after-care rules should be explained to the customer:

1. Always brush wigs with a *wire* brush or *bone* comb. Bristle or nylon help to build up static electricity, making the hair bind on the brush and stretching the fibre.
2. Modacrylic fibres are non-inflammable but will melt if subjected to very high temperatures. Most of them cannot be used with appliances like electric curling tongs, hairdryers or heated rollers *unless thermostatically controlled at low heat.*
3. This type of hair must never be bleached, coloured or permed.
4. Hair lacquer should never be used.

Washing

Wigs should be washed regularly and not allowed to get too dirty. Holding under cold running water will remove surface dust or grime.

For wigs which have been worn a lot, use a special fibre shampoo or ordinary *mild* shampoo with lukewarm water. Rinsing must be thorough, otherwise a film will be left on the hair making it appear dull. These wigs have built-in styling so do not need setting, therefore, hang up to dry out naturally.

* Hints on caring for wigs made from real hair, as opposed to fibre, will be found in the section on Cleaning and Conditioning Hair, on page 72.

Guide to buying

Sheen

A good fibre maintains its natural sheen under artificial lighting or sunlight. Those of an inferior standard tend to glitter under bright lights, although looking fairly natural otherwise.

Shape

A good wig, whether curly or straight, will be shaped well with taper-cut hair. Poorer ones tend to have a bulky look with hair standing away at the neckline.

Texture

Hair texture must feel and look good otherwise the wig will not hold its style. Beware of fibres with a pleasing appearance but which feel coarse. The hair will be springy and hard to control.

Foundation

The wig base or foundation must be well shaped, too, and fit properly everywhere. There should be no undue pressure at any point. It should also be very lightweight, but strongly made. Otherwise it will lose its stretch and become out of shape in a very short time.

Wefting

The hair should be full where it is joined on to the base and the gaps between rows narrow. If not, the base will show through.

Washability

Good fibre wigs wash well. They keep their shape and the hair retains its bounce. Inferior merchandise, on the other hand, quickly becomes limp and shapeless. Also the hair tangles easily and sometimes develops crinkling after washing.

Static Electricity

Inferior fibre hair has the major drawback of a build-up of static-electricity. This causes the hair to be flyaway and impossible to keep in a style. Quality modacrylics do not have this problem.

17 Ready-styled wig in Kanekalon modacrylic fibre.

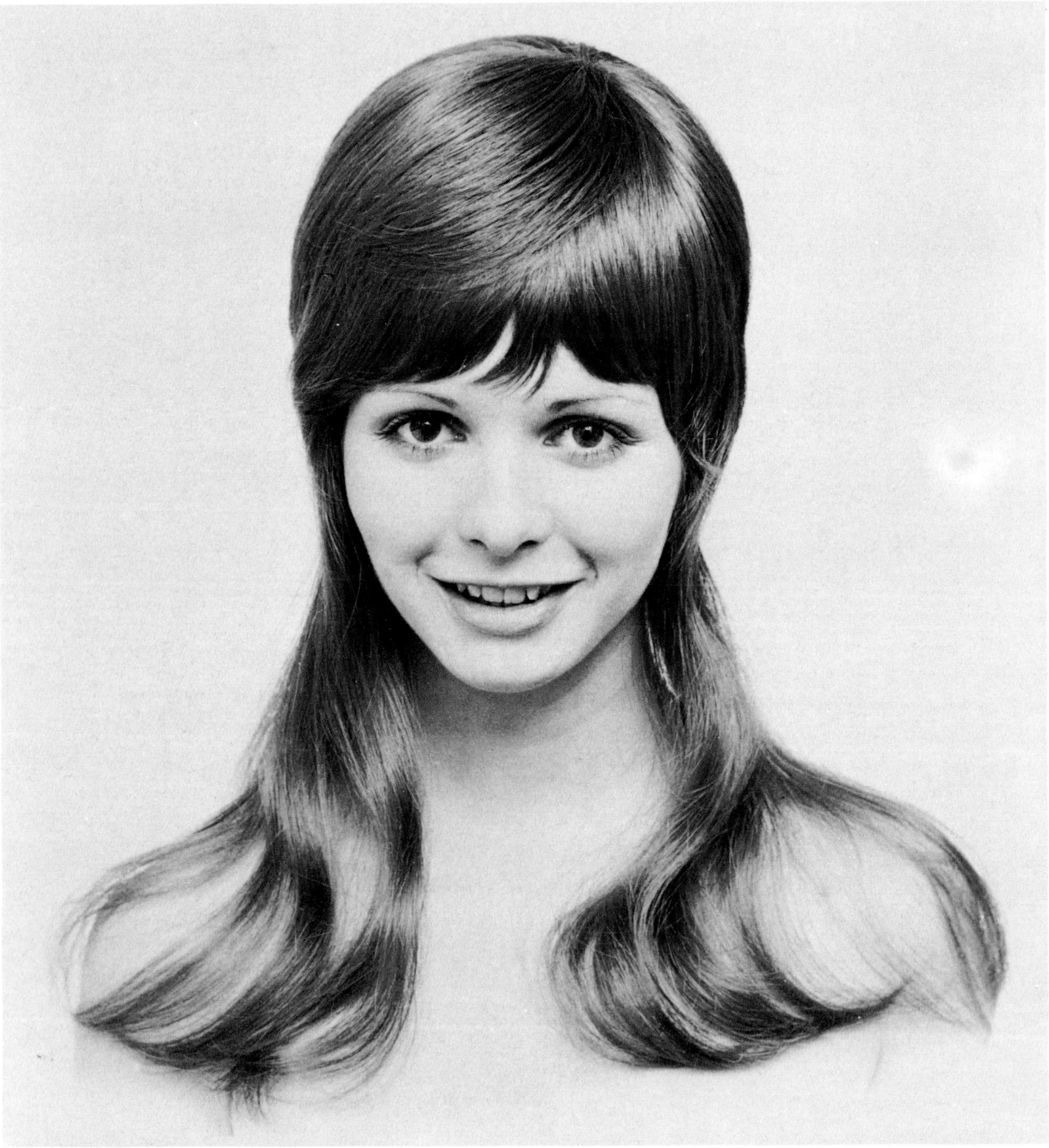

18 Ready-to-wear wig with mixed modacrylic fibre hair.

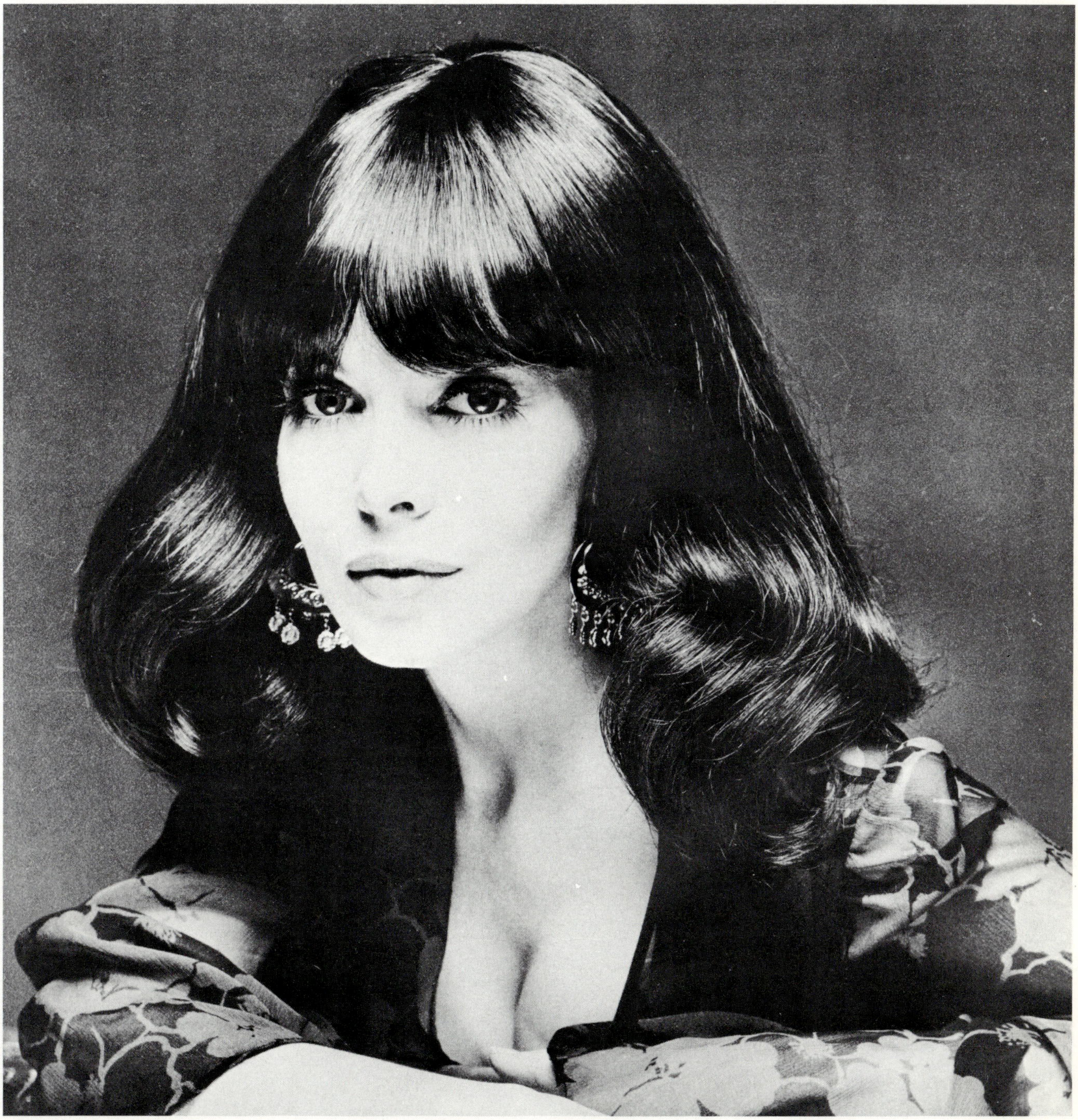

19 Pull-on wig in Dynel modacrylic fibre.

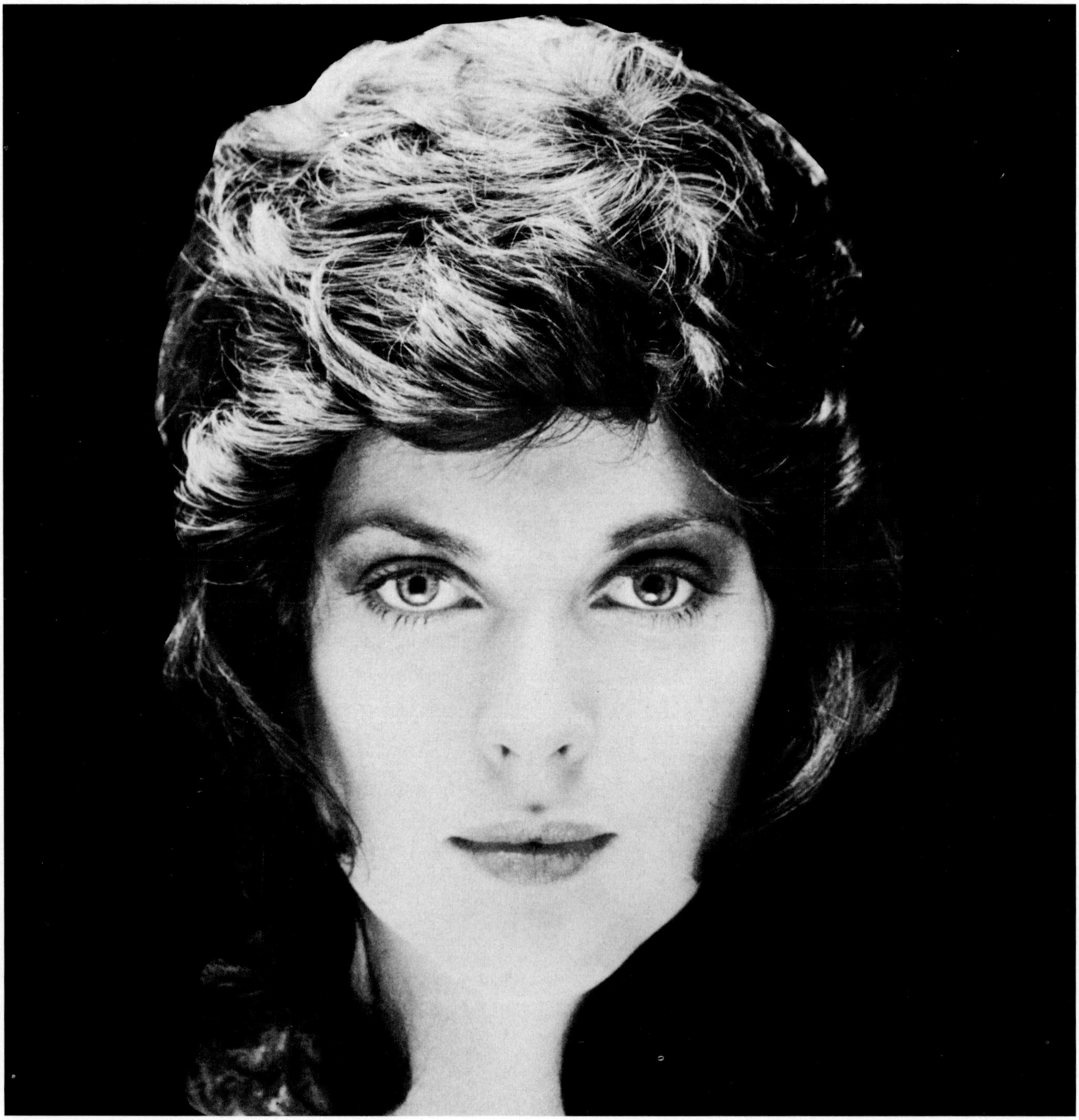

Hair Wigs in the Making

Made-up Asian hair so closely resembles natural hair these days that there is the danger of imagining it will react to colouring, bleaching or perming in the same way as hair growing on a head. It won't though, and this outline of the severe and prolonged processes carried out before it is made up into wigs and hairpieces illustrates why.

The improvement in Asian hair since the first machine-made wigs and hairpieces is considerable. Then it was shiny, wiry, flyaway, and almost impossible to style. Today the best quality is fine, feels and looks very natural, and the pre-permed variety can be styled into any fashionable line. To reach this high degree of refinement it has to be put through heavy and complicated processing because, as already explained, Asians have thicker and coarser hair than Europeans. Oriental hair, also, is either black or very dark brown, which means it has to be bleached and re-dyed to match variations in international hair colours.

First the raw hair, ranging from 10 to 75 cm (4–30 in.) long, is sterilized to kill off any lice eggs. It is plunged into disinfectant and left there for about half a day, then boiled. Later it is put through a knitting hackle to draw the eggs out of the hair, before being rinsed and

20 Wigmaking in Hong Kong started as a shanty industry with hundreds of small one-room factories. Soon large modern factories were designed and built and up-to-date machinery installed.

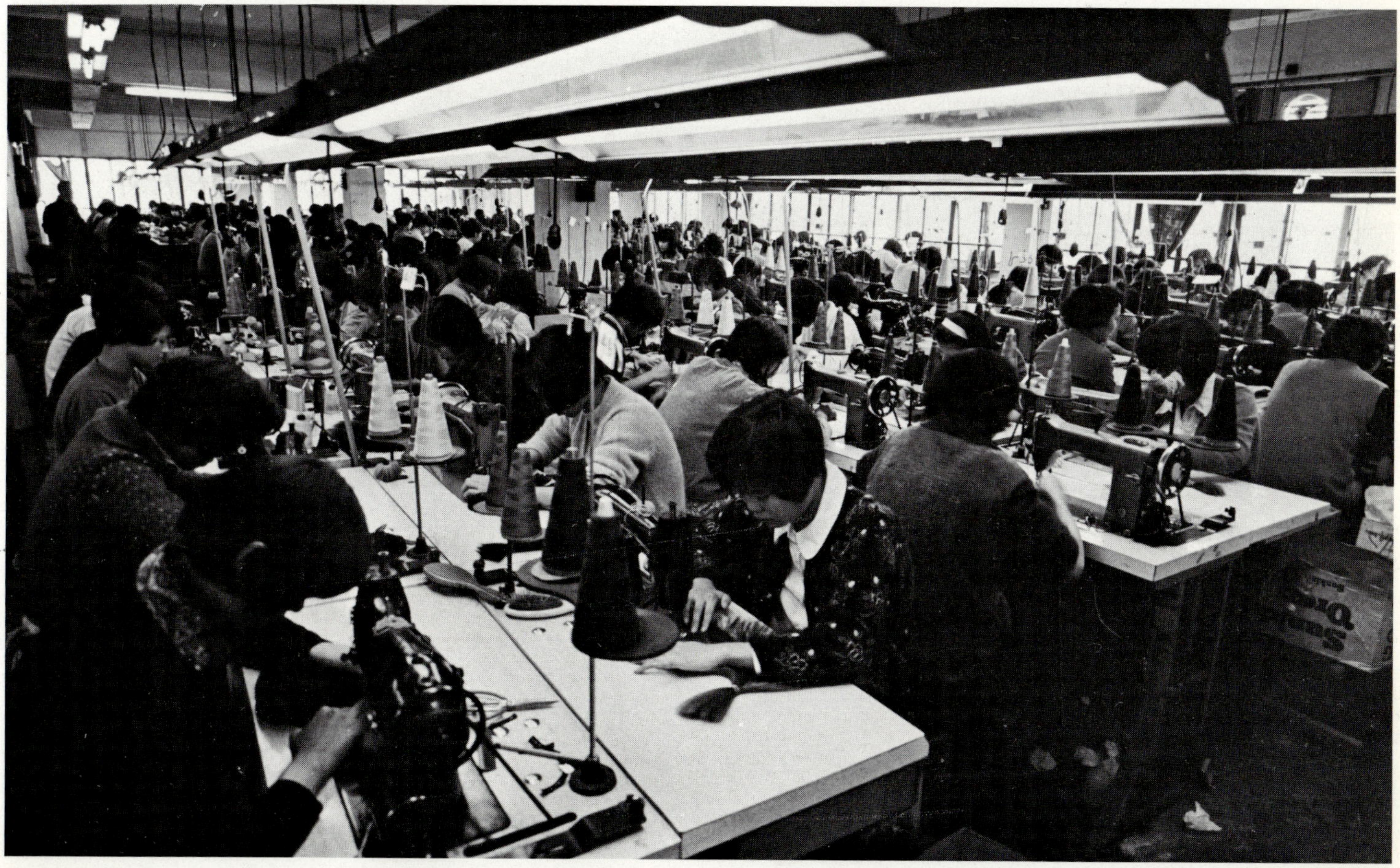

spin-dried. Next comes extensive bleaching. Vats are filled with a mixture of 50-volume hydrogen peroxide, ammonia, and sodium carbonate. In this solution, the hair is boiled for anything up to half a day. By this time the hair should have reached a dark blonde shade. If it has not, the bleach mixture is renewed and the hair left to soak in it for another twelve hours.

This long, harsh treatment strips off most of the hair scales, which has the effect of fining down the hair but also makes it more porous. From the production angle, however, the de-scaling does away with the necessity of sorting the hair into roots and ends.

After bleaching is finished, the hair is rinsed and dried again. Then it is ready for dyeing. The hair is boiled in an industrial textile dye solution (*not* a hair colourant) for up to seven hours, dependent on the shade required. After that, the surplus dye is rinsed out of the hair. Sometimes the hair is put into a chemical softening solution, then dried out again. Next the hair is hackled, sorted into bundles to make it easier to handle, and stored. Later it is weighed before making up. About 115 grams of hair are used for a wig of 10 to $12\frac{1}{2}$ cm (4 oz for a wig of 4–5 in.) and 185 grams for a 35-centimetre one ($6\frac{1}{2}$ oz for a 14-in. wig). Hairpieces take between 55 and 200 grams (2–7 oz).

The bundles of hair, each tied loosely at one end, are dispatched to the machinist. She pulls out the loose ends into a fan shape and machines with a double needle at a slight angle across the hair. This automatically tapers the finished piece. Next she folds over the hair ends into a hem and machines along the edge with a double row of stitching. After that she makes another fold and machines along it in the same way to make sure that the hair will not pull away later. This forms the weft which can be anything up to 360 cm (12 feet) long. Weft for a full wig can be produced in about two minutes by skilled operators.

Finally, this continuous weft is machined on to ready-made wig or hairpiece foundations, made in most cases

21 The raw hair is being put through the first stages of processing—sterilizing followed by bleaching.

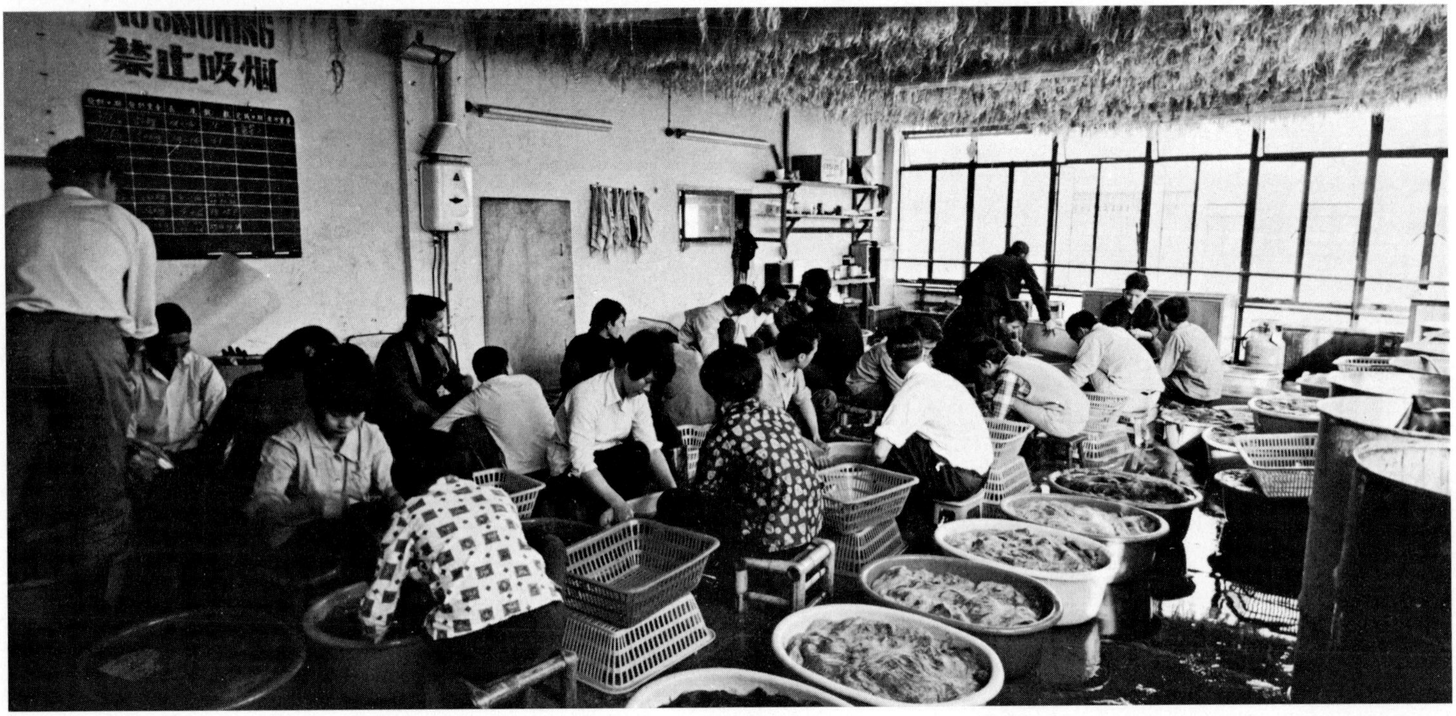

from English net. Some weft is wired and formed into strong bases for longer hairpieces. The better designs are then sent on to another department to be finished with a hand-knotted hairline, parting or crown.

22 (*above*) After dyeing and drying, the hair is drawn through hackles (flat boards with vertical metal teeth). Then it is sorted into easy-to-handle bundles.

23 (*below*) A bundle of hair, tied loosely at one end, is then spread out fanwise and the machinist begins forming the weft. This can be made continuous—any length up to 360 cm (12 ft).

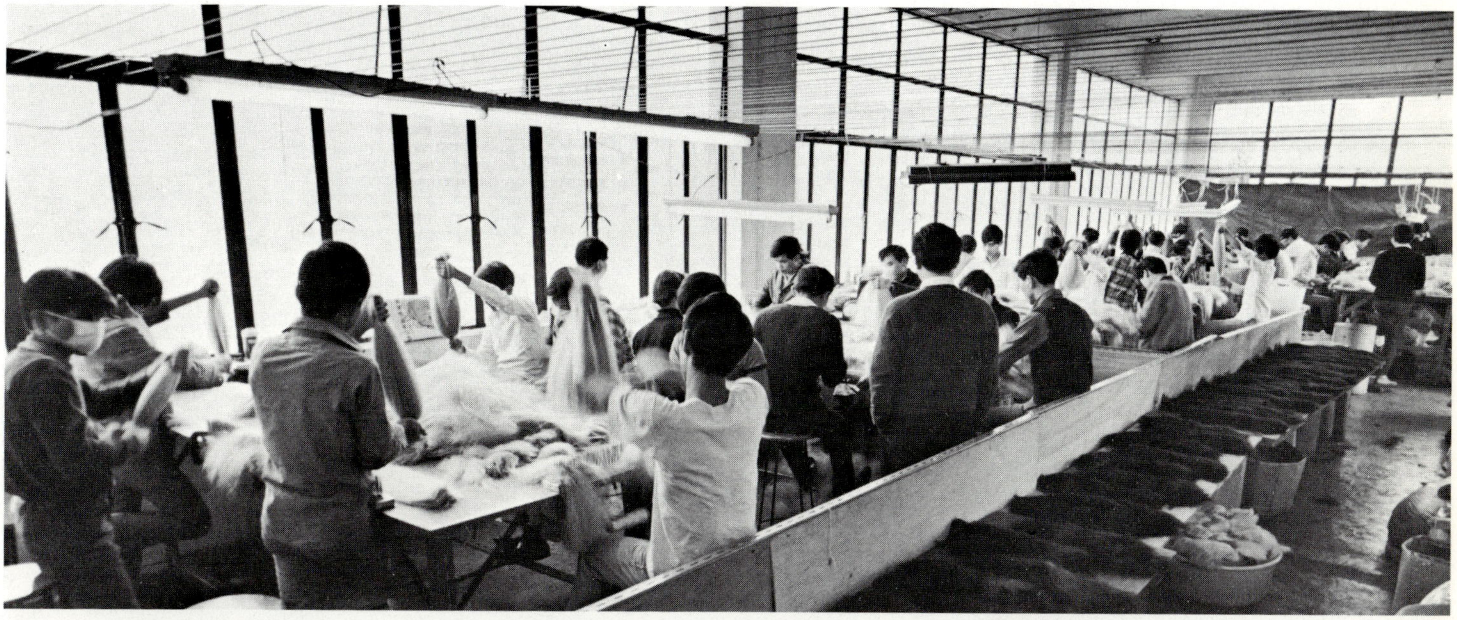

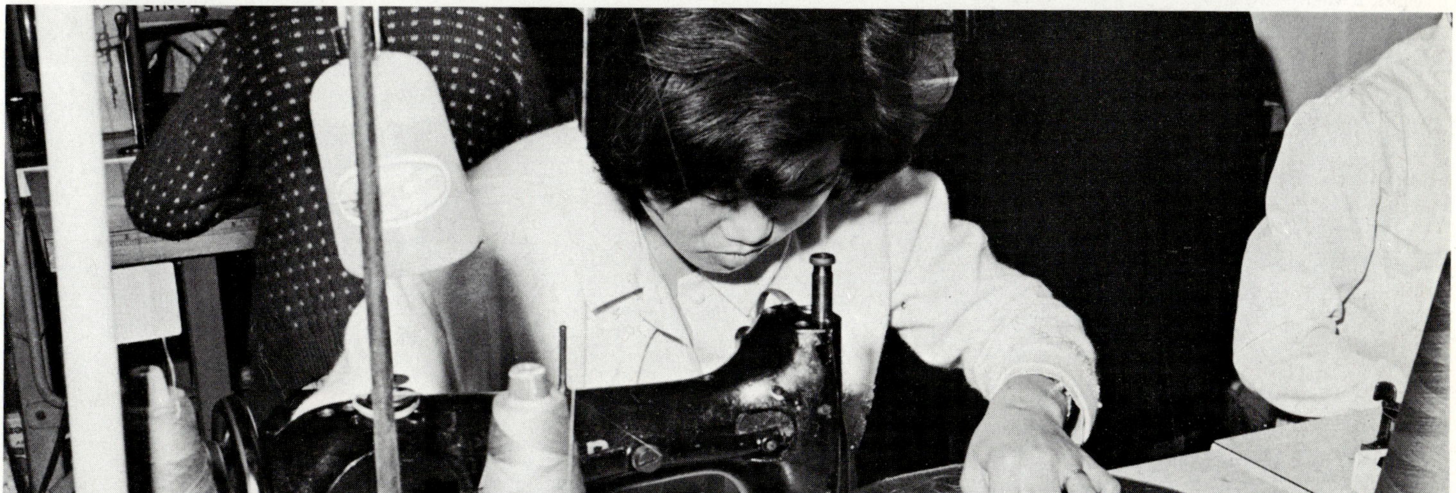

24 (*above*) Some weft is wired, and here is some being made by hand into strong bases to hold the weight of hair on longer hairpieces.

25 (*below*) The better quality wigs or hairpieces go on to the hand-finishing department. There each hair is knotted to the foundation with a fine hook at the hairline, crown or parting.

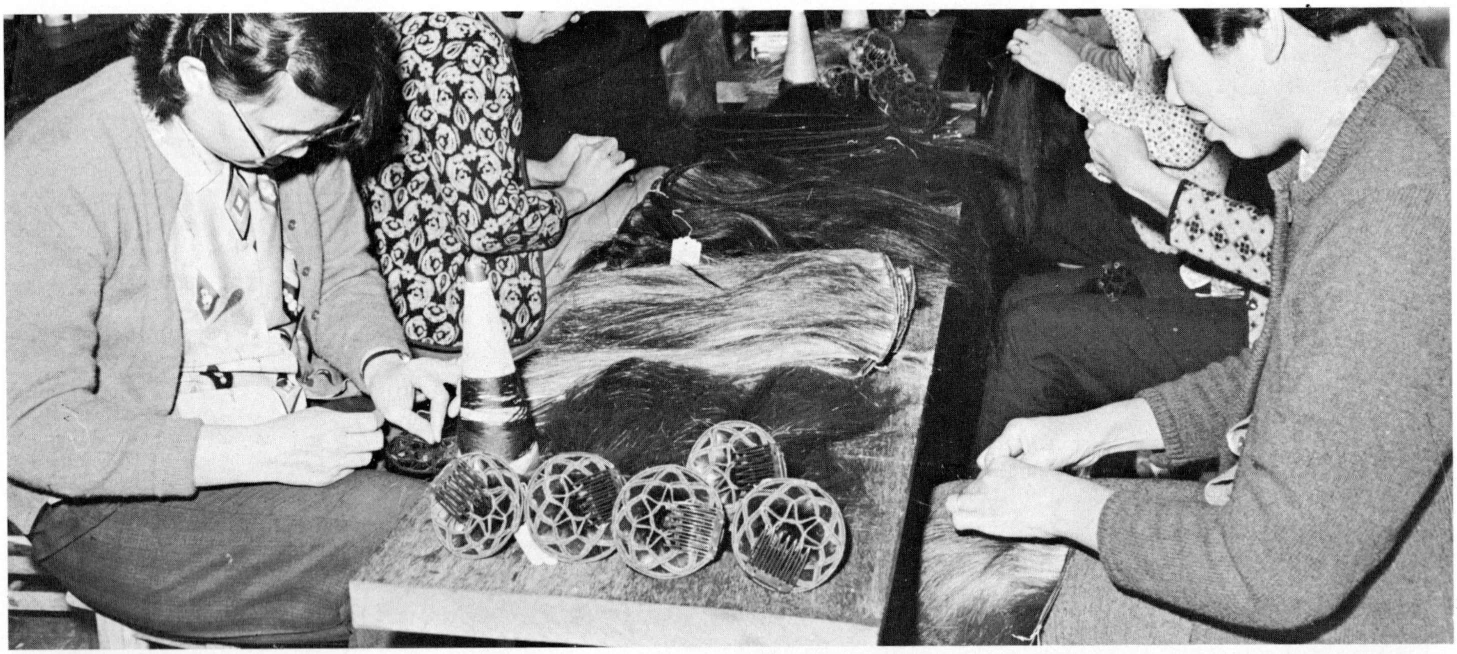

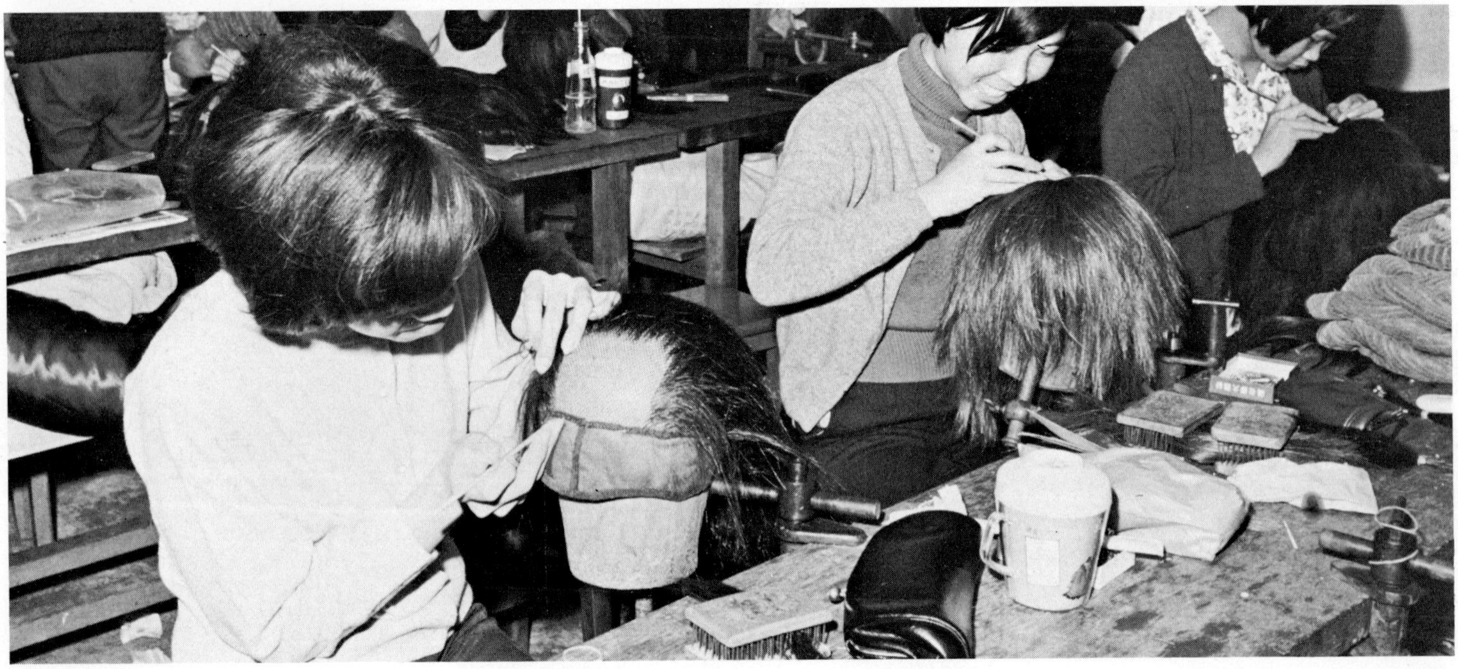

Setting the scene

There's a lot more to the selling operation than salesmanship. Atmosphere, for instance, is equally important for it can start the process of a desire to buy while the person is outside in the street. An impression of specialization and expertise—that's the one to create with this type of merchandise, where the retailer has to play an advisory role. The roots of this particular image lie in an extensive, well-balanced stock plus well-briefed staff with hairstyling flair.

You cannot sell wigs from a catalogue and shade card. Modern woman is impatient and won't wait while a design or colour is ordered—she wants it now! In-depth stock is the only answer and the larger it is, the higher will be the sales. If capital is limited carry the best range you can afford. It is far better to run fewer lines in a good range of colours than to attempt a bit of everything.

Do not get carried away on colours, either. Remember manufacturers' shade ranges for wigs are exceptionally wide, over 100 in fact, but there's no need to try to carry them all. Top-selling colours in this country are the browns; so a full range should be top priority. These, plus a few blonde shades, a selection of greys and frosted mixtures, a black, and an auburn or two, are all that's needed.

Display—a vital factor

It is no good offering a wide range of goods, though, if you fall down on display. A couple of wigs, however elegantly displayed, make no impact whatsoever on the woman in the street; on the other hand, windows packed with wigs of every shape and colour will. The same applies to the inside of the boutique. Every inch of space on . . . walls, dividers, pillars, backs of windows, and shelves should be festooned with wigs. Displays should be constantly changed round, of course.

A good display, though, is not necessarily a seller.

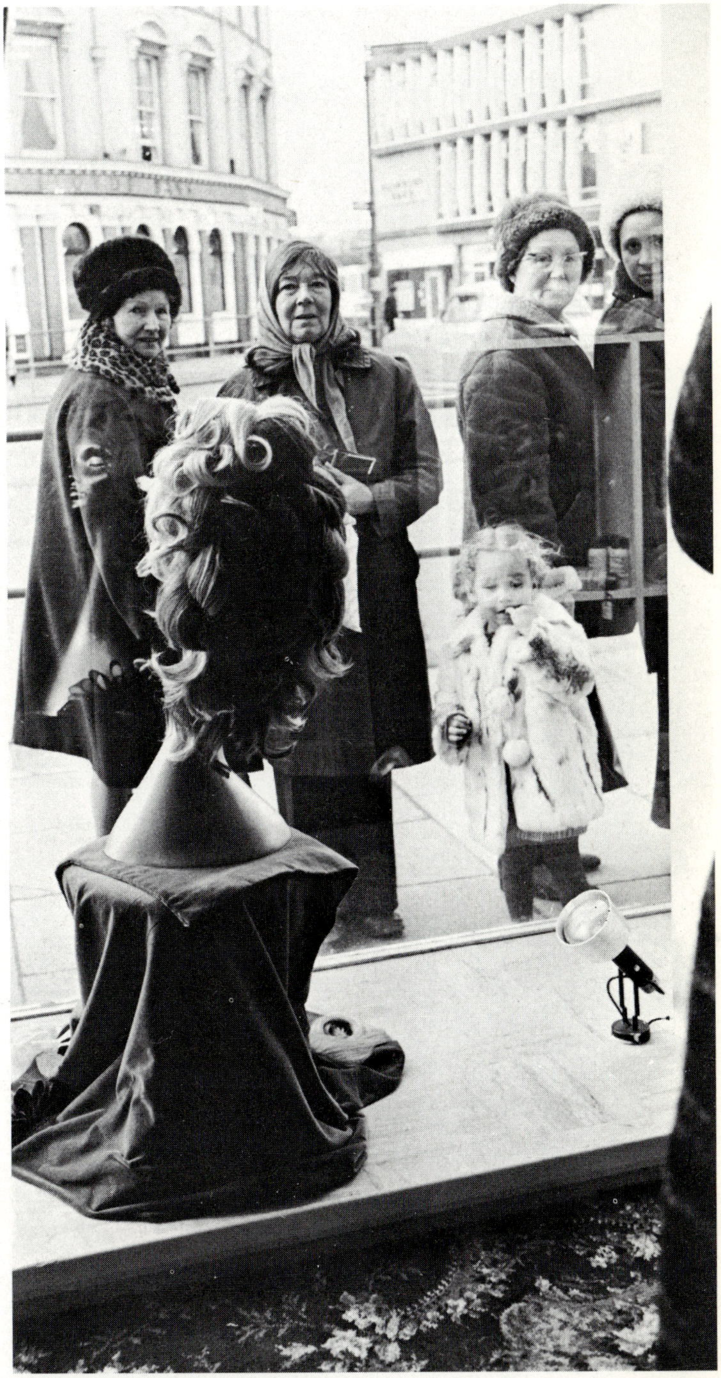

26 Atmosphere and display start creating the desire to buy.

There's one thing, however, that will transform it into one—clear prices on every item. Women are often too timid to come in and ask about prices. Too easily they could assume that your price range was beyond their pocket. So there's nothing to be gained by concealing prices.

Stimulating interest

Once you have set the scene, the next stage is to step up initial interest. Quite the most effective way of doing it is for sales staff to wear wigs or hairpieces, preferably all the time. It attracts a surprising amount of attention from the most unexpected people, and it can be the start of easily-made sales. Another good ploy is arranging for wigs to be brushed out and re-styled near the door or window. This acts as a magnet to passers-by and, again, triggers off enquiries. Oddments marked down in price, heaped in a basket or decorative, floor-standing container, encourage impulse buys. The untidier the heap the better, as women cannot resist turning over the

27 Massed display both in window and interior is a necessity for volume sales.

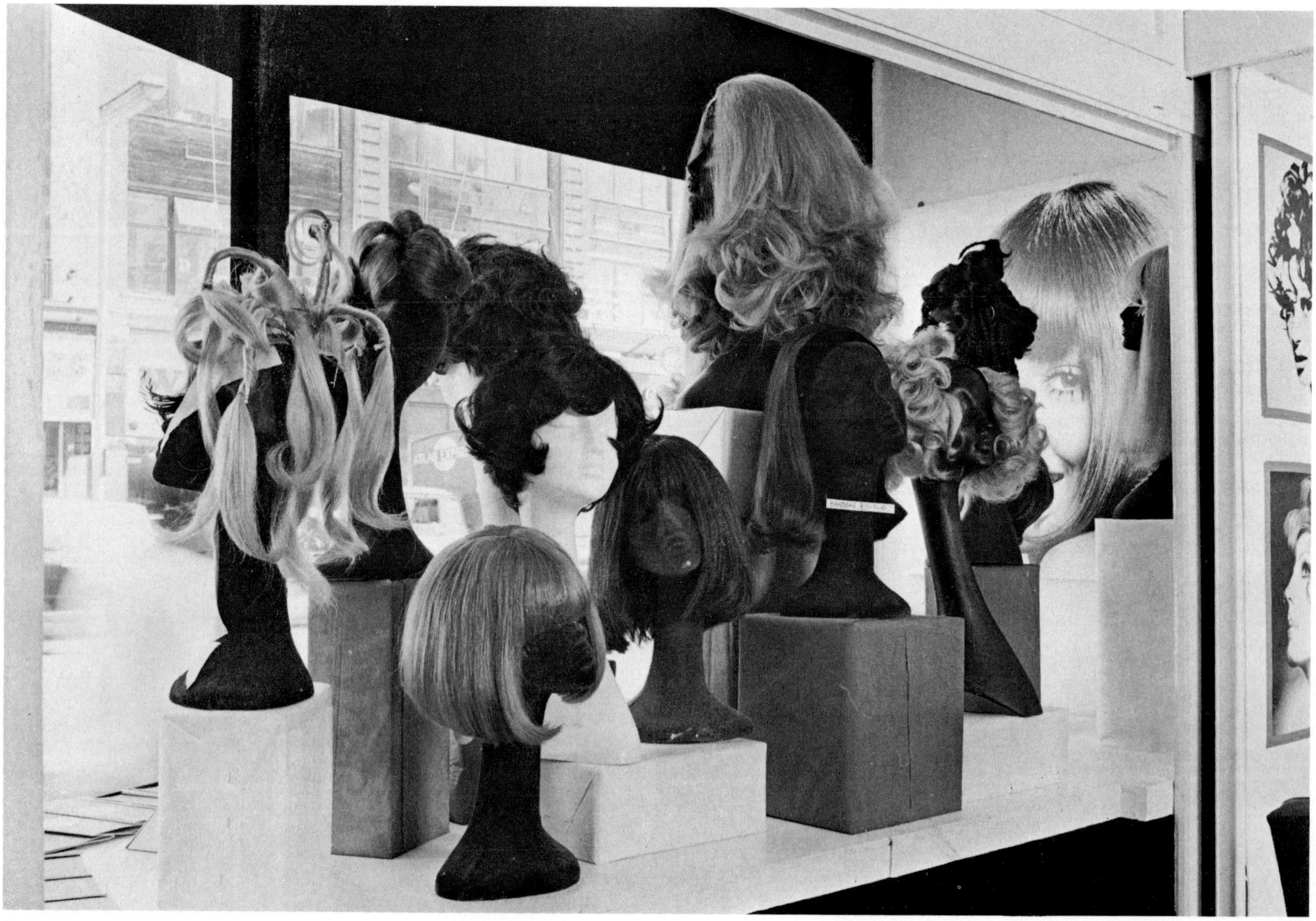

items, convinced that the bargain-of-all-bargains lurks beneath the pile.

A wig trade-in operation, a hire service for bridal or other formal occasions, are also ways of developing interest and stimulating sales. Outside promotions, in the form of wig shows and parties, all help to publicize the goods you sell well beyond the boundaries of your street.

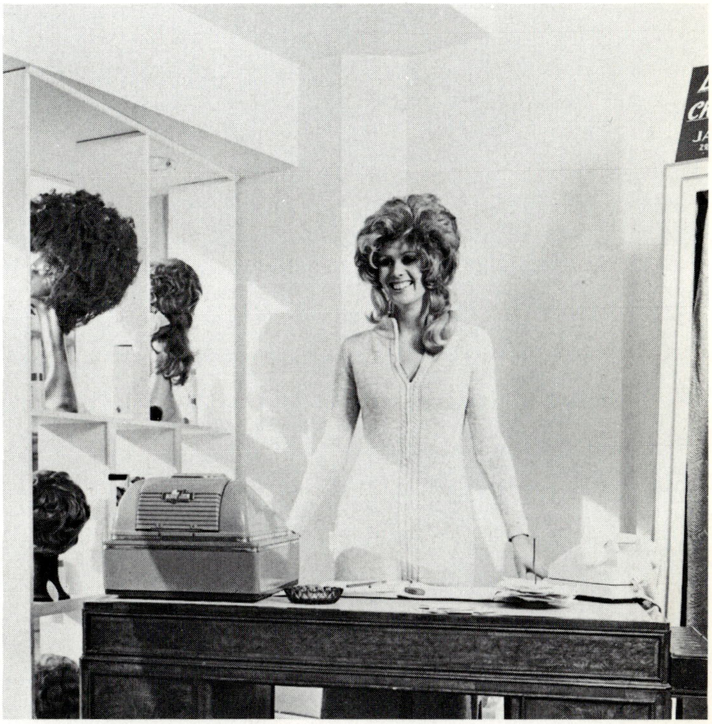

28 Staff wearing wigs or hairpieces attract attention and stimulate interest in added hair.

Basic sales approach

Now over to selling, in which sound product knowledge is the key to success. The more a salesgirl can talk technicalities, the greater the chance of a sale. The selling technique, of course, must be flexible and geared to individual customers. However, whether dealing with a shy or domineering woman, there are four lines of approach to avoid:

a. Lecturing or 'talking down' to her.
b. Ignoring her preferences.
c. Over-selling or pushing too hard.
d. Asking her outright to buy.

Main customer types

Women, of course, vary tremendously but they can be divided into four main customer categories, with basic rules for handling them:

The Muddlehead . . .

Often appears shy with no confidence in her own judgment. Finds it agonizing to choose between more than one article. Asks innumerable questions.

. . . and The Approach

Encourage her and help her to overcome her indecision. Don't show her too many articles to increase her confusion. Give her all the technical information she wants, she'll listen eagerly. Put to her leading questions needing 'yes' for an answer, like: 'Now you can see why I think this wig would suit you best don't you Madam?'

The Slowcoach . . .

Usually walks and talks deliberately and takes endless time to decide to part with money. Never make the mistake of assuming that she is stupid, though.

. . . and The Approach

Nothing will rush her into making a decision so extra patience and sustained interest are necessary. Allow her plenty of time to absorb each sales point, which should be re-phrased and repeated until there is some response.

The Know-it-all . . .

Usually a strong character who likes airing her knowledge. Often infuriating but she's not necessarily just trying to be difficult. She merely knows exactly what she wants.

. . . and The Approach

Compliment her by commenting on her knowledge but never allow yourself to appear intimidated by it. Avoid disagreeing with her at all costs and call in a senior if necessary.

The Wordless One . . .

One of the trickiest to handle, as she shows little reaction to the usual sales 'leads'. Often ignores or fails to answer questions. Should not be assumed to be dim-witted, though.

. . . and The Approach

Show extra friendliness and interest. Try to make her feel at ease. Keep up a gentle flow of talk, but no waffling! Lead her into handling the merchandise. Put questions that need the answer 'yes'.

Arousing the desire to own

Once a customer shows more than a passing interest in a wig, making her want to own one is the next step. Here the approach should begin with involvement. Persuade her to feel the texture of the hair . . . the lightness of the wig . . .the firm construction of the foundation. At the same time, question her indirectly about the kind of life she leads and the type of social activities. Then assess the best kind of designs for her needs. Ask indirect questions such as:
'Has it ever struck you, Madam, how much time a wig can save you?'
'Did you realize, Madam, that a wig can save you money you'd spend on hairdressing?'

Then move on to the advisory role producing several designs to look at. Make comparisons and stress that you have chosen the selection specially for her—and why. A curly style to soften her features . . . a new colour to accentuate her eyes . . . or a more elaborate design for her special occasion. Make sure that it all leads up to making her want to try them on, for once she has reached that stage, you are well on the way to making a sale.

Closing the sale

After leading the customer to the brink of buying, then the sale has to be clinched. This, the most vital stage of all, is often assumed to be the most difficult. It isn't once the initial fear of talking a customer into buying has been overcome. After all, the signs of mounting desire to own are easily recognizable. Every time she answers in the affirmative to indirect questioning, she is moving nearer to buying. Then is the time to move in and lead her gently towards making a decision, with statements like:
'I think you'd need the wig styled to your face Madam. I could start on it right away, if you like.'
'Perhaps you'd prefer a little less hair at the sides. Should I go ahead and have the wig thinned out for you, then, Madam?'
'Don't you think it would suit you a bit shorter Madam? It would be no trouble to thin it out for you right away.'

There are endless variations, of course, but the basic selling technique remains the same; gentle persuasion all along the line combined with a strong advisory role.

Follow-up profits

There is a tendency to be content with making a sale and thinking no further than that. Profits, however, need not end there, for there is a great potential in wig after-care. Follow-up servicing such as cleaning, conditioning, and setting, and with hair, colouring and perming as well, can be built up into a regular and highly profitable side of the business. This can either be carried out in the boutique with hairdresser-trained staff or farmed out to a nearby hairdressing salon. The clever way to make a quick start is to book the customer for an after-care appointment the minute she has bought a wig!

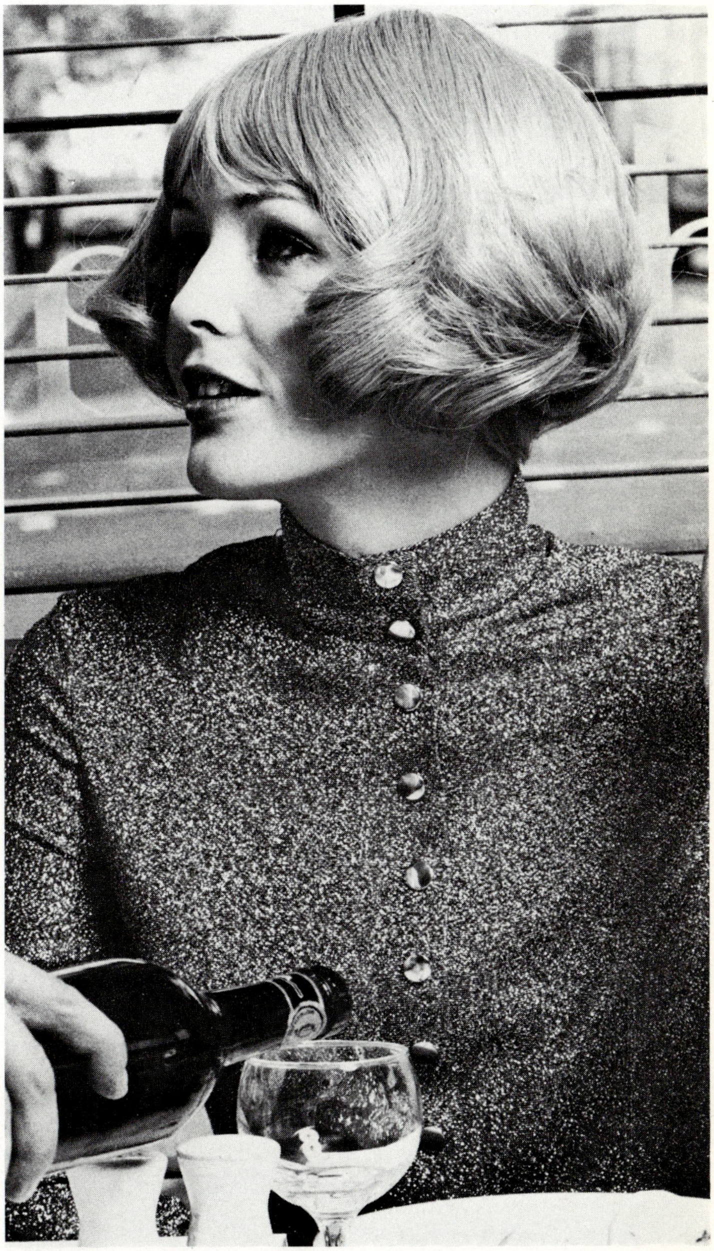

29 Getting your wigs talked about outside the boutique is important.

Everyday Promotion

Beyond the boutique

There are still a great many women who do not own a wig, so the potential is still enormous. If capturing a substantial slice of the market, though, is your aim, constant and effective promotion is essential. There is a lot that can be done without spending vast sums of money.

Displays in window and interior are fine but not enough for really thriving sales. In every locality there are places outside the boutique where you can arrange for wigs to be displayed.

For instance, what about a fashion shop? There could be a two-way tie up. You could add glamour to your displays by showing their merchandise. They, in return, could put wigs among their fashion clothes. In many towns, too, there are showcases in various places—hotel lobbies, office block entrances, car showrooms, etc. These are ideal for 'spreading the message' about your wigs.

Then there are the fashion shows at department stores. All the models taking part in those should be wearing wigs supplied by you in return for a credit on the programme. Do not forget the women's clubs and organizations either. They make extremely receptive audiences for wig shows, so do the women's services or wives at military camps.

Finally there are your local newspapers. Keep them informed of the wig shows you are staging or any other promotional plans. They are always looking for news and you can end up with a lot of invaluable free publicity.

Seasonal theme

Wigs to take on holiday, is an excellent seasonal promotion theme to help boost sales. Special displays, backed by wig parties or shows, built around this idea can lead to volume sales. 'Planning a holiday? Then you'll need a wig to cover up that sea-drenched hair' should be the motto. Getting the message across to women's organizations or clubs with a female membership should be the aim.

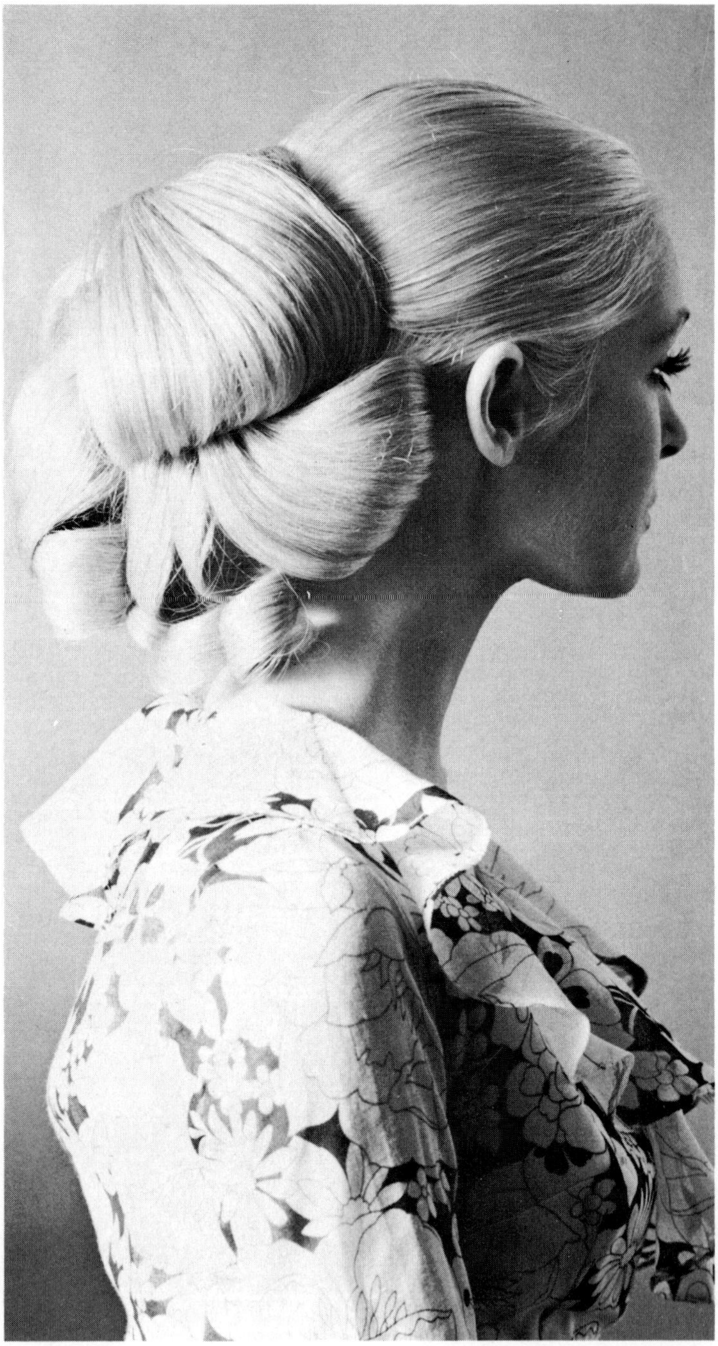

30 Models in local fashion shows should be wearing your hairpieces or wigs.

Before working out details of the show, consult your wig supplier first. Some will lend stock for the event on a sale-or-return basis. Often, too, they will arrange for a representative to be present, if the show is large

31 Sun and sea play havoc with hair. All the more reason for a holiday wig.

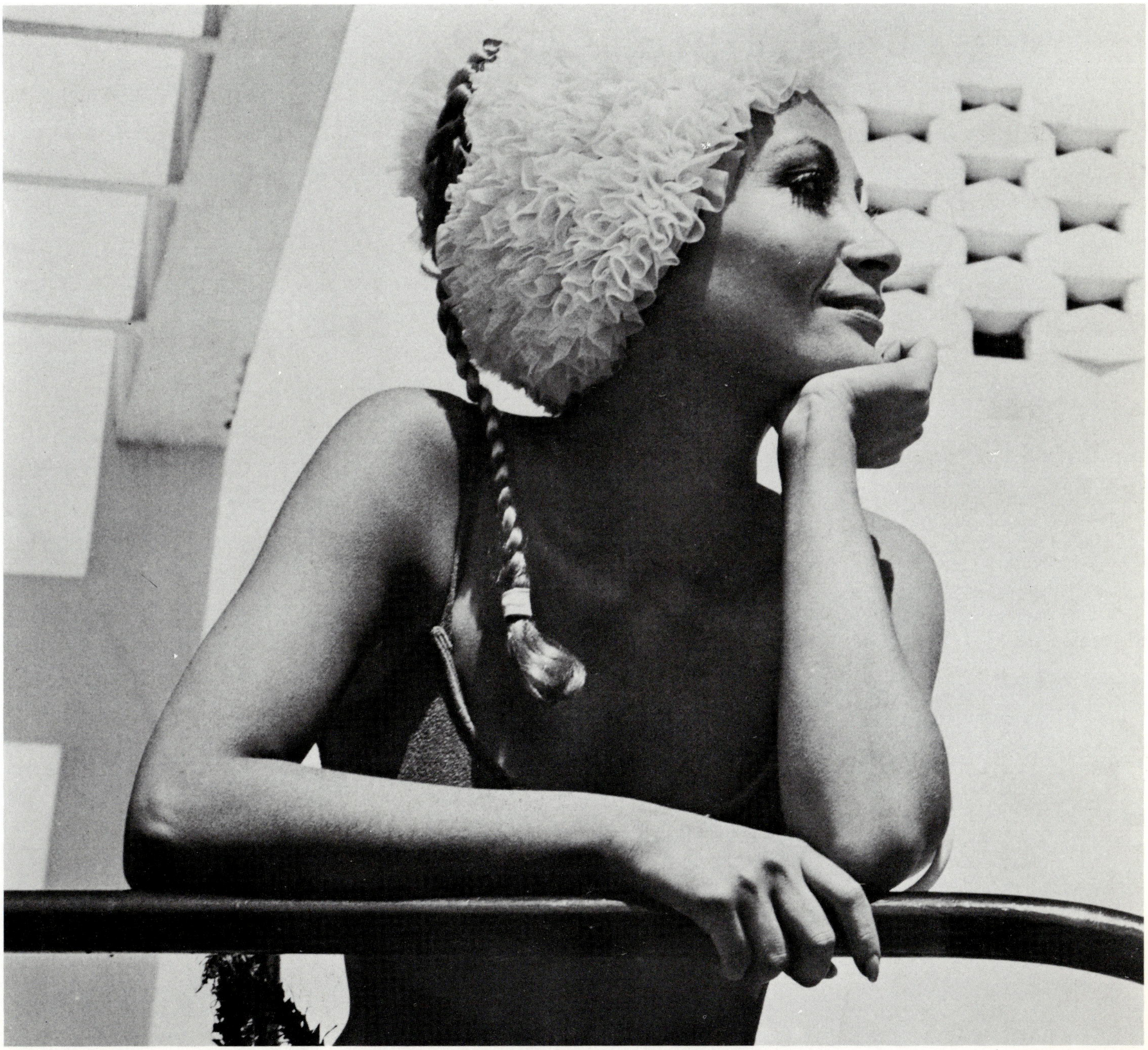

enough to warrant it. When choosing the designs to promote, put the accent on simplicity. No holidaymaker wants to spend hours arranging a wig. So confine yourself to well-cut, natural looking wigs and demonstrate

32 Natural looking fibre designs which can be brushed quickly into shape are good for holiday promotion.

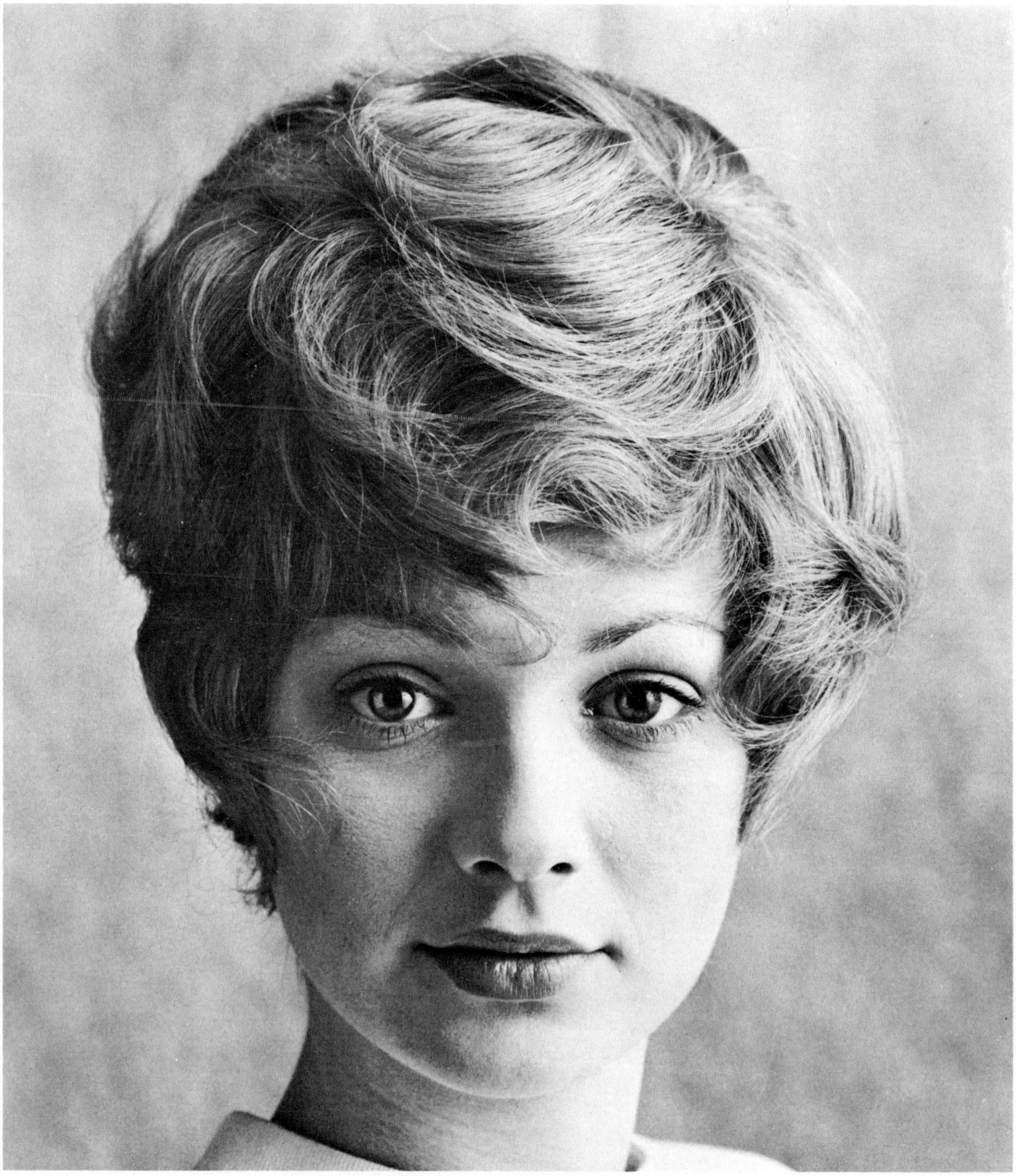

how they can be arranged in a variety of different styles.

Do not limit the holiday range to fibre wigs, either. Some women will prefer hair on the basis of going 'one better' than their neighbours. Make a big feature of the

33 Some customers will prefer a hair wig to take away with them.

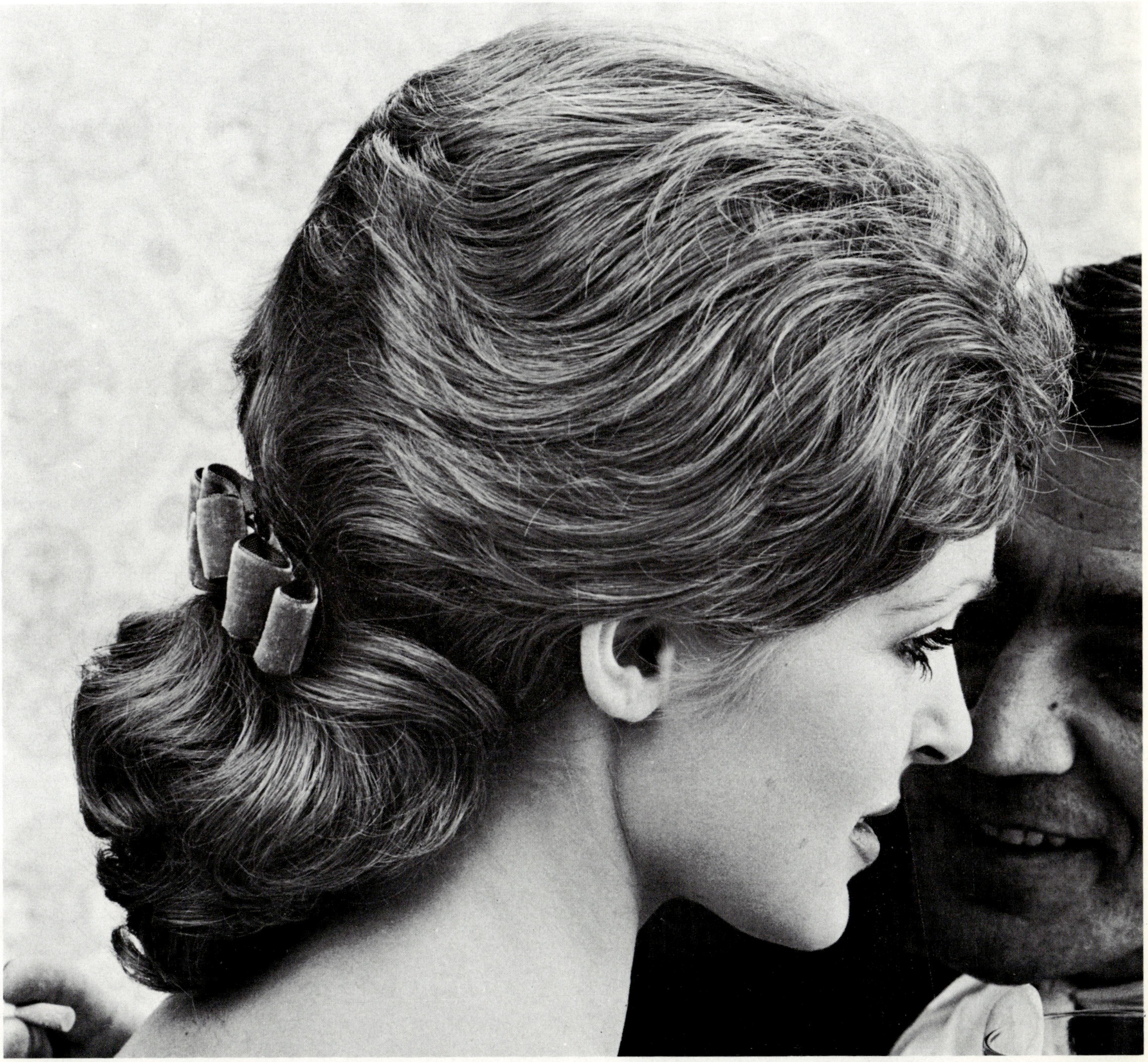

frosted and highlighted shades. They look particularly spectacular teamed with colourful beach clothes. A 'wigs only' show is too narrow a concept. Introduce fashion clothes and accessories to broaden the scope. Emphasize the holiday message with things borrowed from local fashion shops or boutiques.

Let the models carry gaily coloured beach bags and holdalls or giant beach balls or blow-up toys. Have them wear . . . sunglasses, headbands, bows and ponytail clips or other hair ornaments, swimcaps, scarves, beach hats, and ponchos or tabards. You can always put them on sale afterwards.

Also do not overlook wig accessories as an extension to sales. Arrange an attractive display of spray-on wig cleaners or conditioners, shampoos for fibre wigs, wig heads and cases, or heated roller sets. If you want to take it a step further, group the goods in a smart beach holdall. Call them 'holiday wig care packs', and run them as a series of special offers during the show.

Now back to basic planning. Another important aspect of the show is the commentary. This must be lively and non-stop. Remember, to keep up chitchat for half-an-hour or more requires a tremendous number of words, far more than you would suppose. Therefore, take no chances. Get down to some homework beforehand and work out a script so that you can keep it running all the time.

To make it interesting and informative your commentary should include the following points—all of which can be developed from information given in this book: (An historical background to wigs appears on page 37.)

1. Wigs throughout history—and the role of the posticheur.
2. The rapid growth of the fashion wig industry.
3. The major wig fibres and different types of hair. Sources of supply, properties, and uses of each.
4. The intense processing through which raw Asian hair is put before being made up into wigs.
5. A detailed account of manufacturing methods in wig factories.
6. Cleaning and general care of wigs, both hair and fibre. How to prolong their life and wearability.
7. Introduction of the idea of a wig wardrobe, pinpointing the appropriate designs to cover any social or other type of occasion.

Always leave plenty of time for a trying-on session. Remember, however, it will need careful organizing or it can easily get out of hand. Arrange to have as many assistants there as possible to control and speed things up. Another girl should be put in charge of sales and order-taking. Give her a section by herself, well away from the trying-on area. Be prepared to sell more wigs than you expect and top up your stock well beforehand!

Publicize the show in the window, as well as inside the hairdressing salon or wig boutique, offering, of course, free tickets within. Send announcements to all the women's clubs in your district, too, not forgetting teenage and youth clubs. Postcards in newsagents shops is another cheap way of publicizing the event. And if you plan to advertise in the local newspapers, do so well in advance. This will enable you to revise your plans and find a larger hall should the applications for tickets prove overwhelming—something which invariably happens!

These, then, are the ingredients for a successful promotion. Combine them with an imaginative approach and you are all set to cash in on the holiday season and boost your profits on wigs.

Practical slant

Do not be content with pushing wigs merely as instant glamour. Look around for other reasons to promote them as well. The obvious one, of course, is thinning hair. Though what about the do-it-yourself hairdressing blunders like . . . frizzy perms, ragged cutting, breaking hair caused by over-bleaching or garish streaky colour effects? These go on all the time and there are plenty of women cringing from the sight of ruined hair. Put across the idea of a wig as an instant cover-up and they will be your friends, and customers, for life!

Preliminary presentation

It is fatal to take a wig out of its plastic bag and put it straight on an older, shyer customer's head. Her first horrified reaction will be how ludicrous she looks. If you tried, you couldn't find a better way to kill a sale! You may not realize it, but nothing looks worse to the non-expert than a wig before it is brushed out or partially styled. You can envisage the final flattering

34 Wigs can be pushed for reasons other than instant glamour.

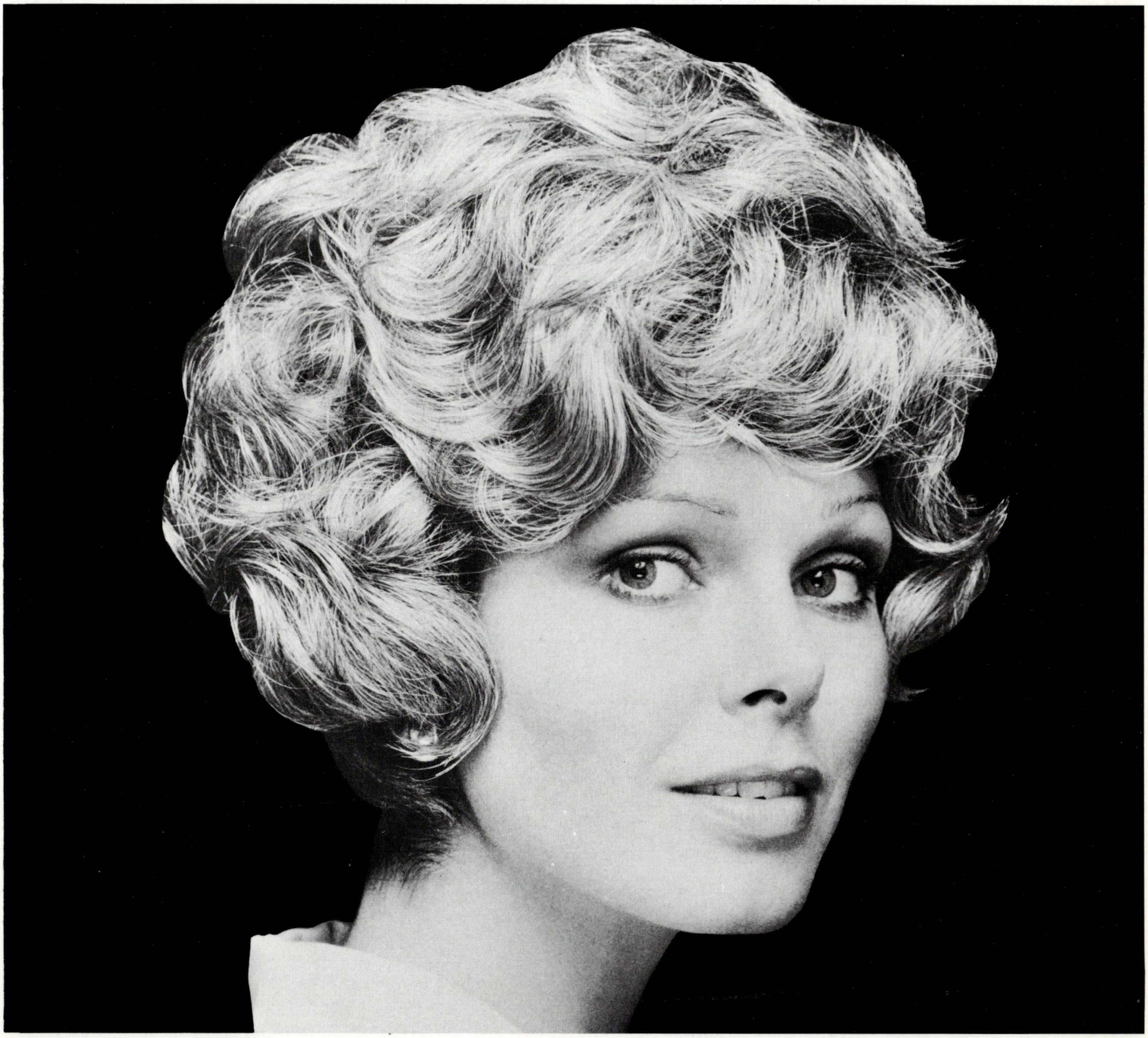

effect. The new customer cannot. So make a new No. 1 rule. *Never* have an un-dressed wig anywhere it can be seen by the public. The same applies to wigs or hair-pieces which are being cleaned or re-styled. All servicing work should be banished behind the scenes. Stained wig blocks or limp, straggling hair can destroy the glamour image of a wig for ever.

35 Greater care must be taken when presenting a wig to an older customer.

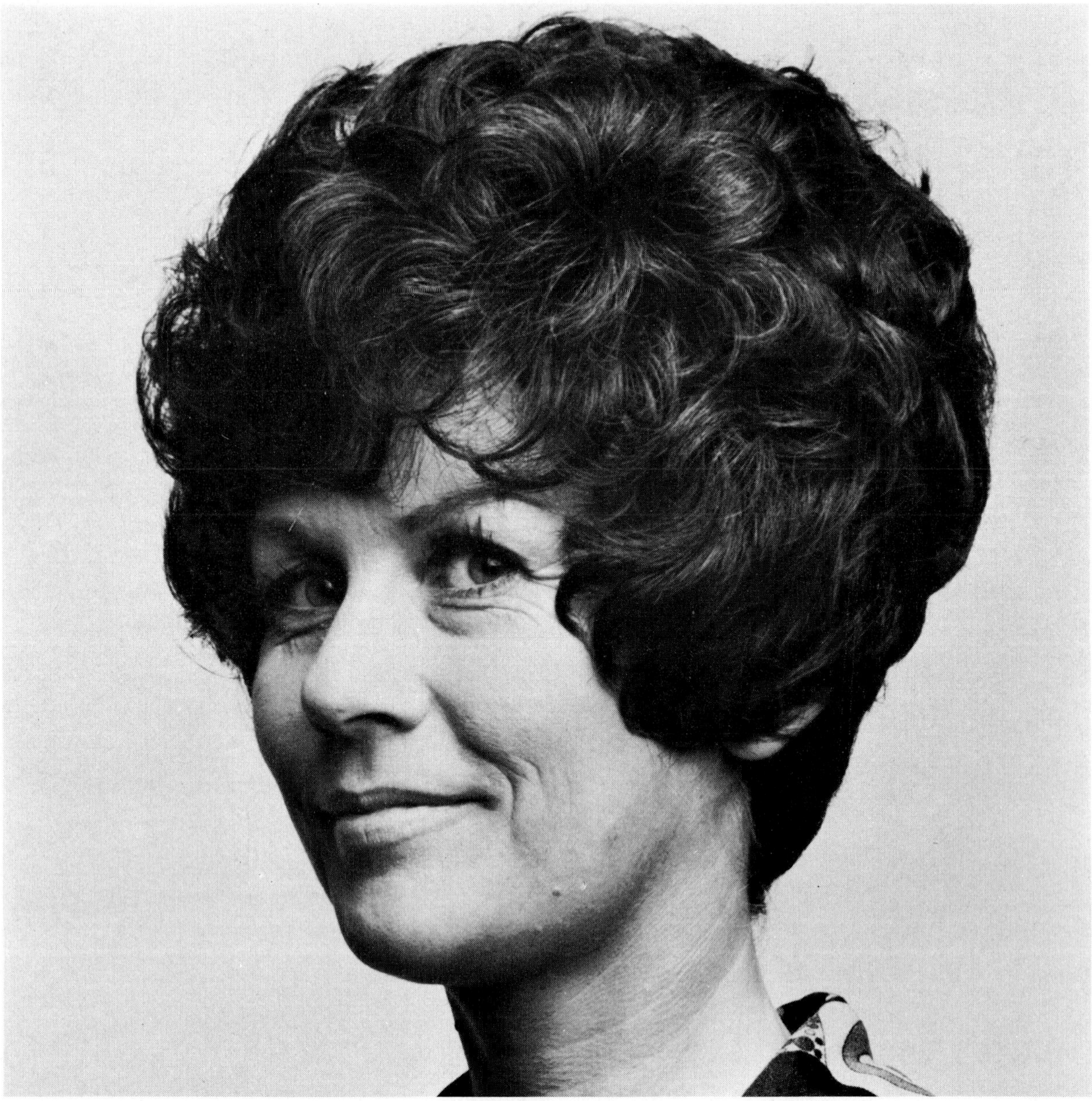

Added Hair Through the Ages

Background for wig show commentaries

There is nothing new about the concept of wigs and hairpieces. From early Egypt to the present day, wigs or cunningly concealed false hair have played their part in fashionable hairdressing. So today's vogue for wigs is merely history repeating itself. The Egyptians revered wigs. They wore them as symbols of social status. The Roman matrons went in for them, as well, to cover up hair they ruined by bleaching with lime! They knew a thing about quality, too. Their wigs were made from German slavegirls' hair. Even today hair from European sources is accepted as the best in the world for wigmaking.

Up to the 1500s, hair was mostly dressed as a foundation for headdresses. Halfway through the century, however, frizzing and back-combing came in. Hairstyles became high and elaborate and false hair was used to achieve it. Hair was gummed into all kinds of fantasy shapes and then powdered, presumably to cover up the gum. About that period, false ringlets or curls were called wigs and a complete head of false hair was known as a periwig or peruke.

By the beginning of the 1600s, ruffs and crimped hair were in vogue. These tightly curled hairstyles were uncomfortable, though. So much so that women took to having their heads shaved and wore periwigs instead. Wig-wearing eventually faded out of fashion at the time of the French Revolution. After that, false fronts, fringes, long curls, and chignons were used to create a studied *déshabillé* effect.

Wide false braids followed and hair continued to be dressed elaborately until the early 1900s. By then the young were having short cuts and taking to perming and Marcel waving. This, of course, brought about a dwindling demand for transformation pieces, except from older women with thinning hair.

The Victorian and Edwardian ladies concealed the fact that they wore false hair. They hoarded their hair combings to make pads for chignons, buns or high piled curls, made up for them by the hairdresser or posticheur. The false hair was sorted and then drawn through a hackle (a flat board with metal teeth sticking upwards) to straighten it. Hackling, incidentally, is still used today, both for blending raw hair or removing tangles from made-up wigs.

Next came the job of sorting it into bundles with each hair lying in the same direction. This, as you can imagine, was slow and tedious, requiring a great deal of patience. Finally the hair was sorted into lengths of 7½ cm (3 in.) upwards, ready to be made up into false pieces. Sometimes the hair had to be curled. Wood or hardened clay, shaped sticks called 'bigoudis' were used for this. Sections of hair were rolled up on these sticks and then dropped into boiling water with a touch of soda. The sticks were boiled for several hours, then taken out and dried in a warm atmosphere or in an oven for extra speed. The dry hair was then unwound and stored.

This stick method of curling is attributed to the Egyptians. They used to plaster their hair with river mud, as a kind of setting lotion, and roll it up on to sticks. The women then sat in the sun while the mud dried and then combed it out of their hair.

Shade mixing was, and still is today, a very important part of wigmaking, requiring a great deal of experience plus an accurate eye for colour. This is especially important for top-quality wigs, as several shades are blended together in a close resemblance to natural hair which always consists of a mixture of shades. In those days, the posticheur or wig specialist often re-coloured the cheaper wigs with vegetable dyes, or even tea or coffee. Metal was sometimes added to produce darker shades. Eventually, special dyes used for furs were found to be ideal.

So the false hair story continued until the early 1960s when mass-produced wigs and hairpieces burst upon the world. From then on, all former reticence about wearing false hair quickly disappeared.

Hand-wigmaking still flourishes, however, and is part of the recognized training of a hairdresser. The technique is admirably covered in the *Manual of Wigmaking* by Mary Botham and L. Sharrad (Heinemann). Untouched by competition from the machine-made variety, handmade wigs are still very important.

Basics for Beginners

Blocking

Although the majority of foundations are now made of stretch material, there are variations in size and shape. Therefore, it is essential to fix a wig on a correct sized, malleable block before cutting, cleaning, colouring or perming. If the block is too large it will over-stretch the foundation, or encourage it to shrink if too small. A malleable block is shaped to denote the back of the head and has a centre seam to be used as a marker. Pinning must always be done with special T-shaped postiche pins, designed to hold the wig firmly while work is in progress. Cover the block with clear plastic sheeting to protect it from process solutions.

See Figures 36 to 38 on following pages.

Setting hair

First block the wig. Then thoroughly wet the hair with cold water or setting lotion but do *not* saturate the foundation. Stagger the sections of hair to be put into rollers. That prevents the foundation from showing through when the hair is styled. Wind the hair on to smooth metal rollers, not the brush variety which easily get caught up into this type of hair. Be careful not to buckle the hair ends when winding. Secure each roller with a T-pin. Pincurls and hair which is just brushed into shape should be anchored with T-pins too. Then put the wig under a hot hairdryer for up to four hours. Allow the hair to cool before styling it.

See Figure 39.

Measuring for length

Personalized cutting, or cutting to suit a customer's face, requires careful planning. As the major part of the cutting will be done on a block, guidelines for length must first be made on the customer's own hair and measurements taken from there.

See Figures 40 and 41.

36 First place the centre seam of the foundation on the block seam. Half-insert a T-pin, taking care not to pierce the foundation fibres.

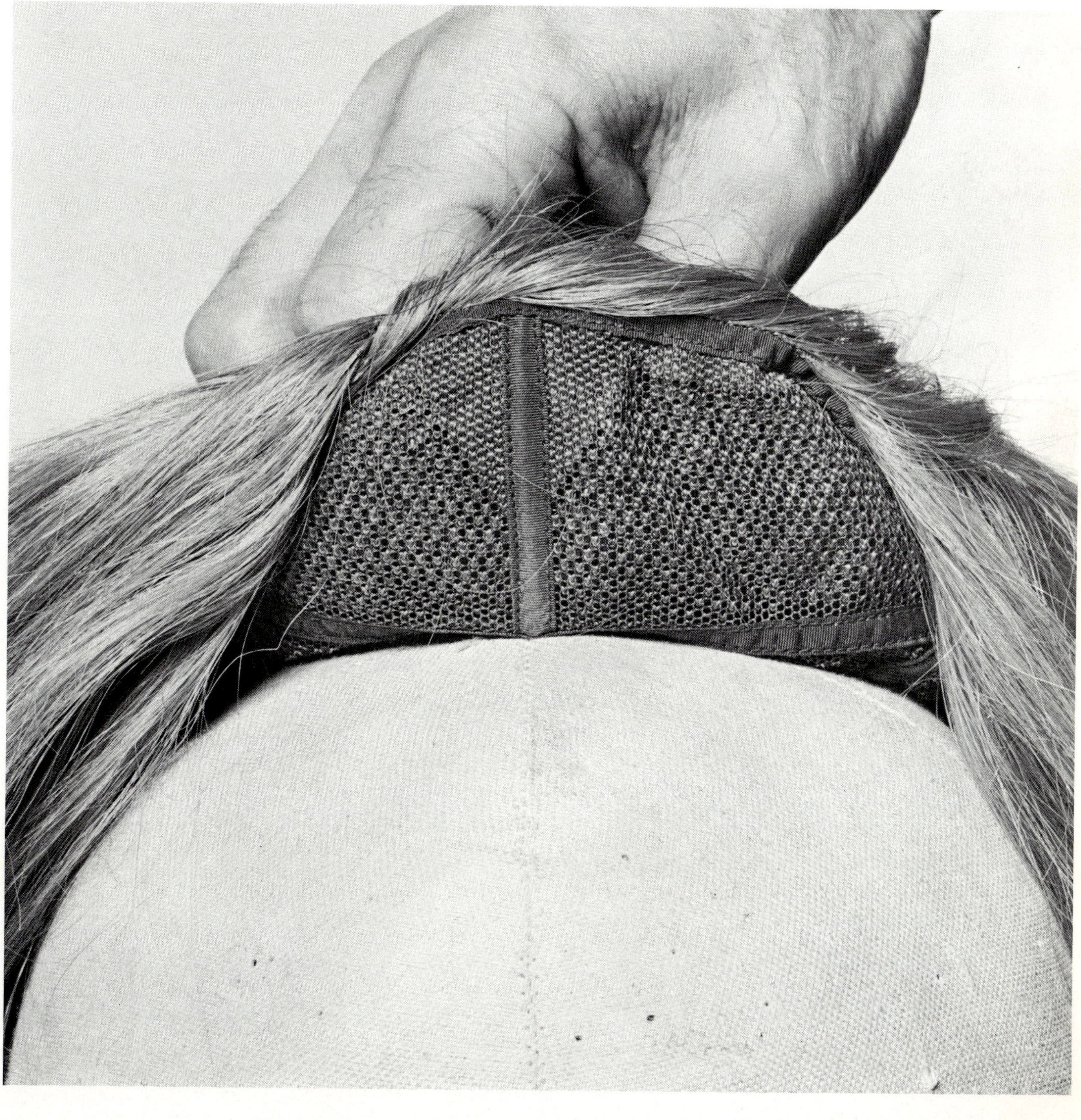

37 Next pull down the sides of the wig and half-insert a T-pin into each. It is important to make sure the foundation edge lies completely flat against the block.

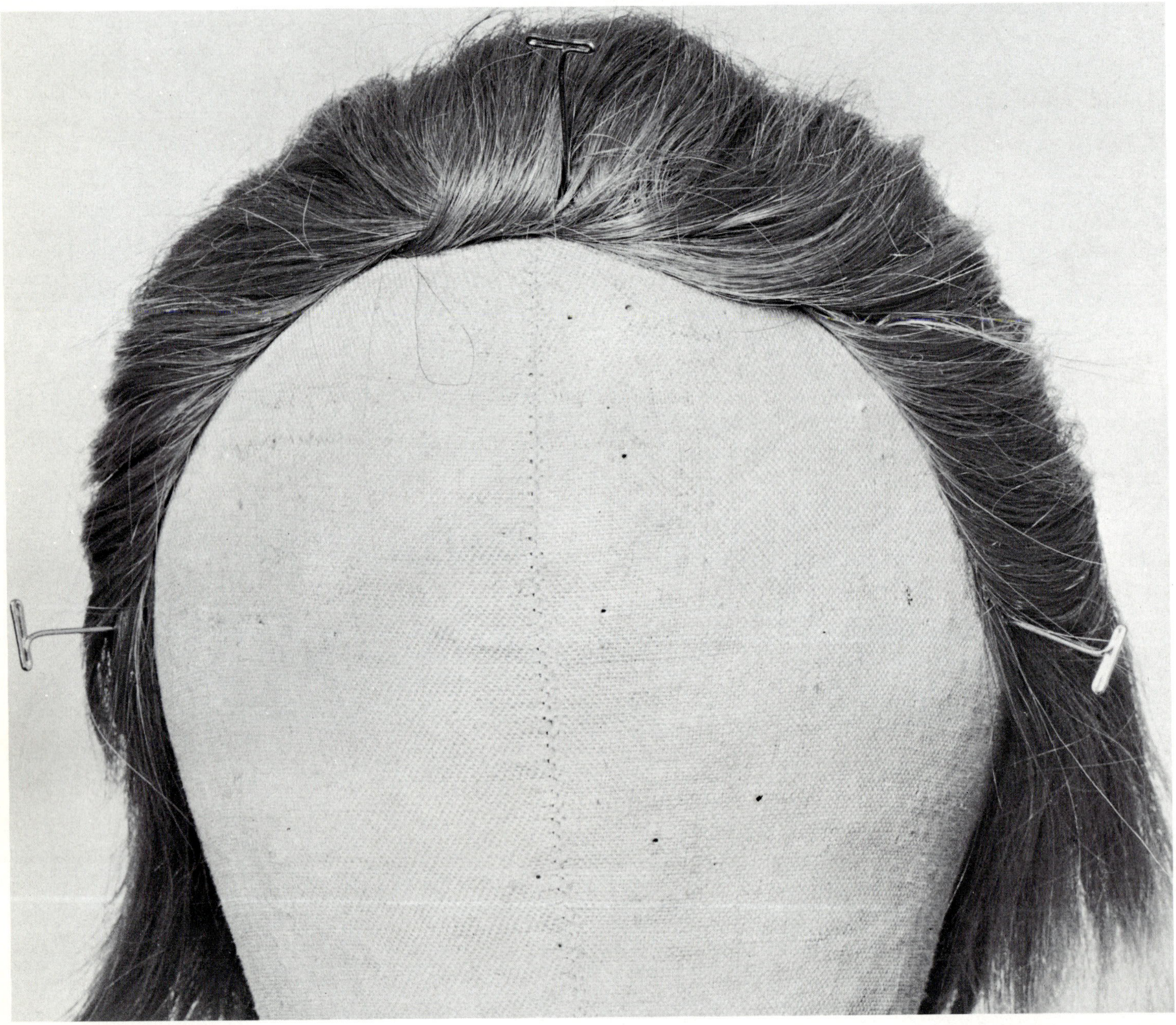

38 Pull the wig down firmly over the back of the block and insert a T-pin at centre nape. Then put in two more T-pins—one on either side. Finally push all the pins right down into the block until they are firmly embedded in it.

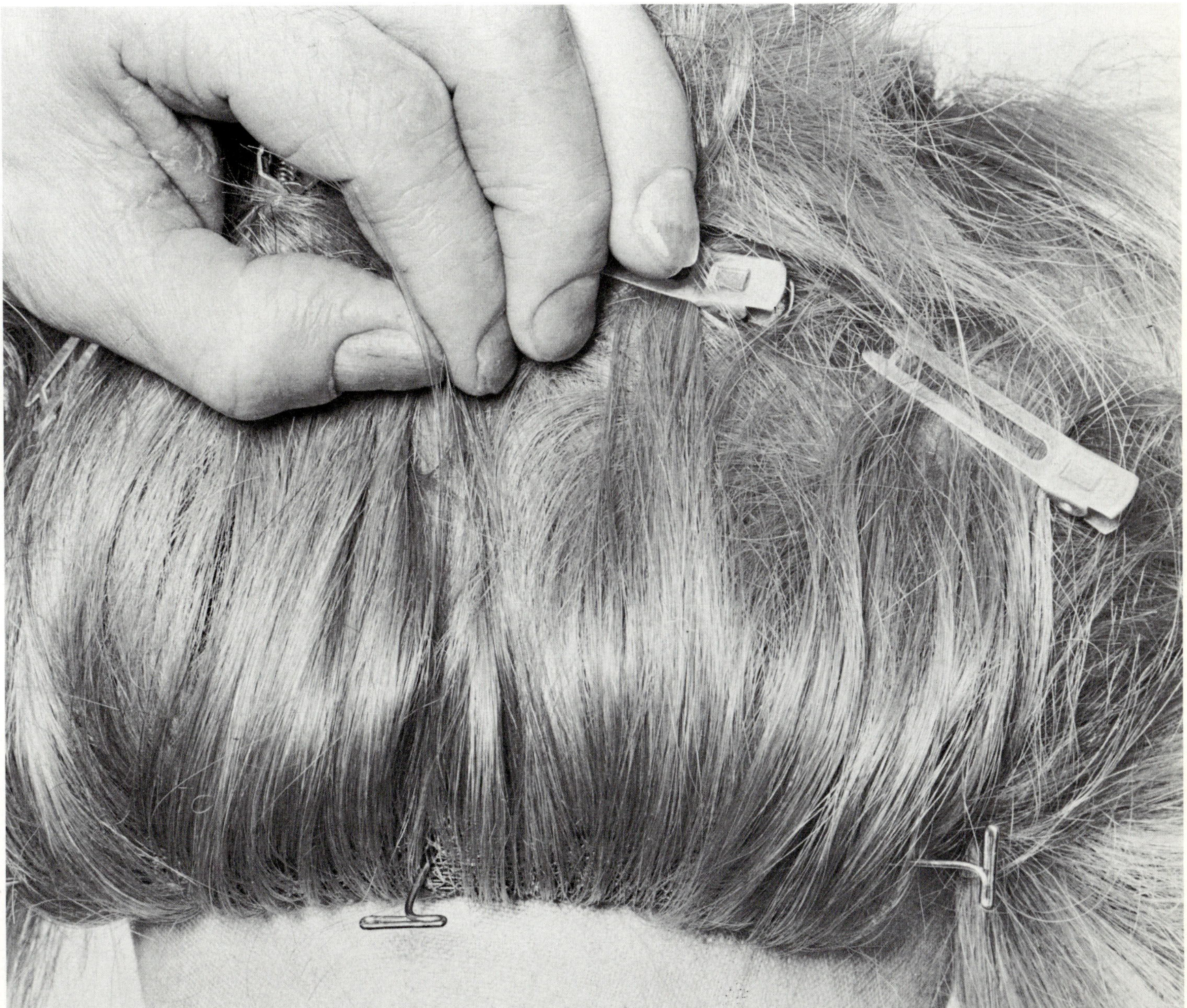

39 Setting hair.

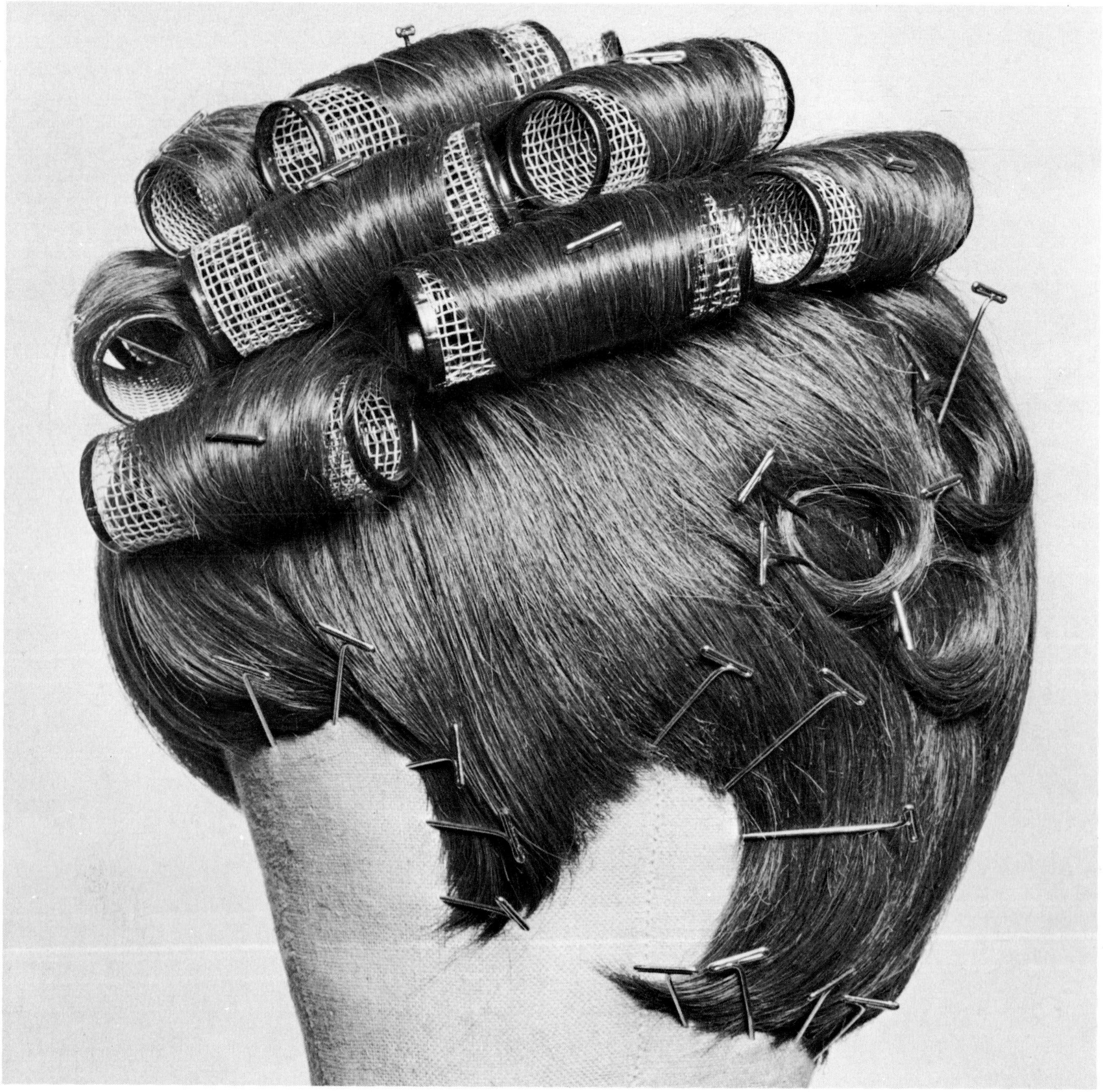

40 First try the wig on the customer to check fit. Then remove and block it until you are ready to start cutting. Return to the customer's hair and decide on the length the wig is to be. Measure and mark with a cutting at the front and sides . . .

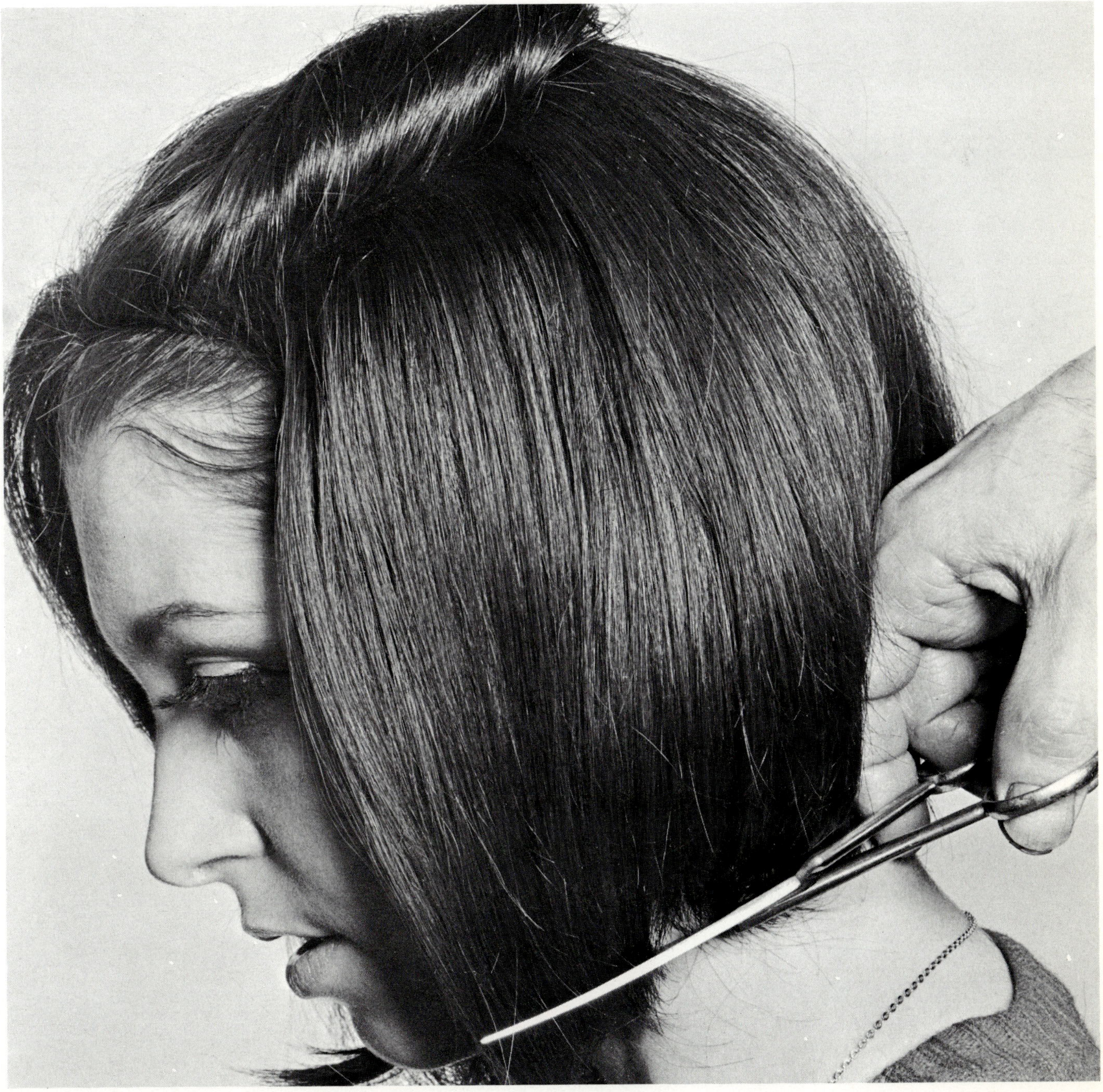

41 . . . and again at nape centre. These points are then your guide for cutting the wig. (A step-by-step demonstration of professional cutting appears on pages 52–63 and 68–71.)

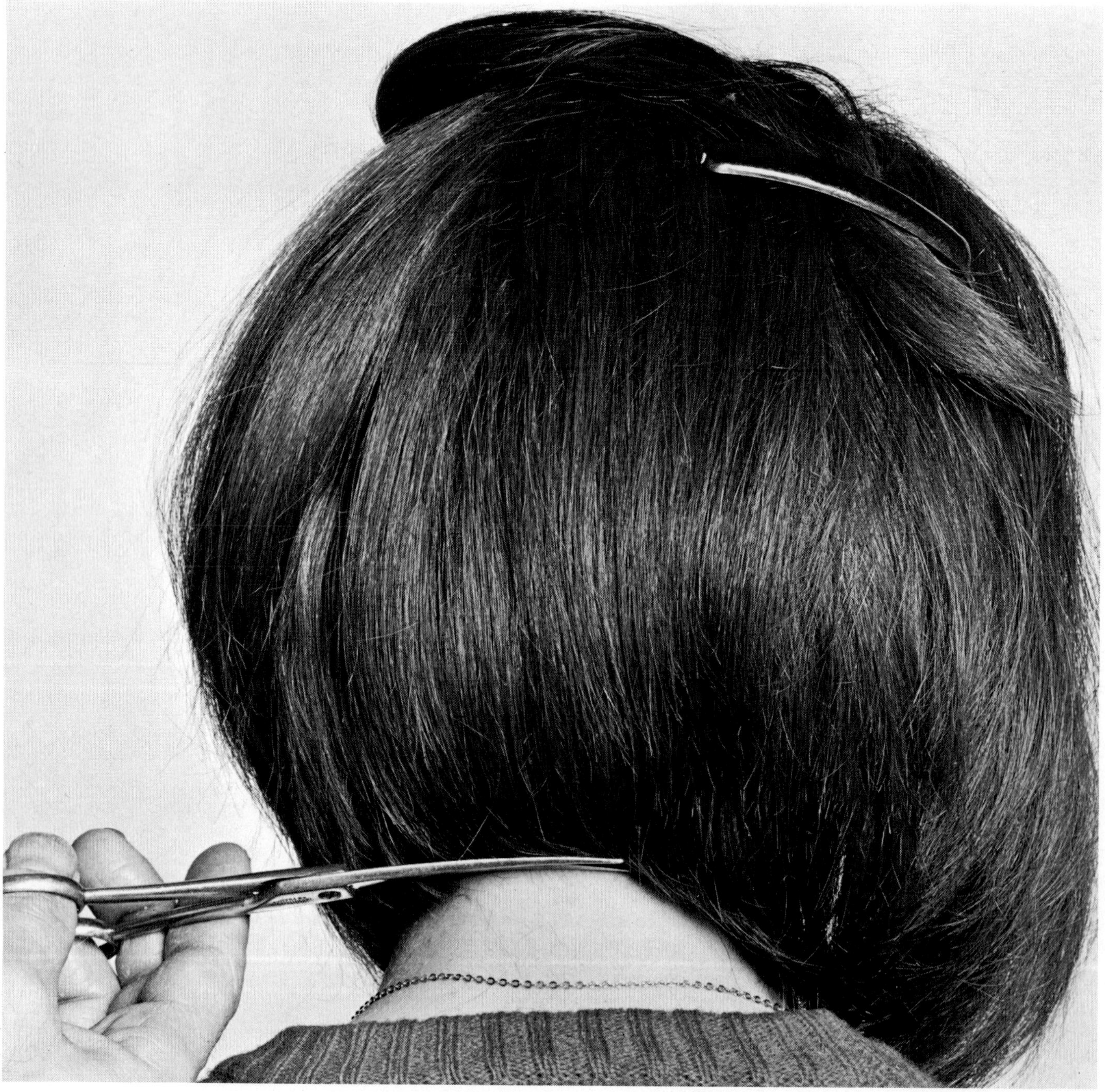

Fixing and fitting

Positioning a Hairpiece . . .

42 First decide on the hairpiece position. Then, from that spot take a section of the customer's own hair, 4 cm ($1\frac{1}{2}$ in.) square. Back-comb the hair if it is very fine and form into a pincurl. Anchor with crossed hairgrips. (If the piece has a very large base make two pincurls side by side with the same overall width as the base.)

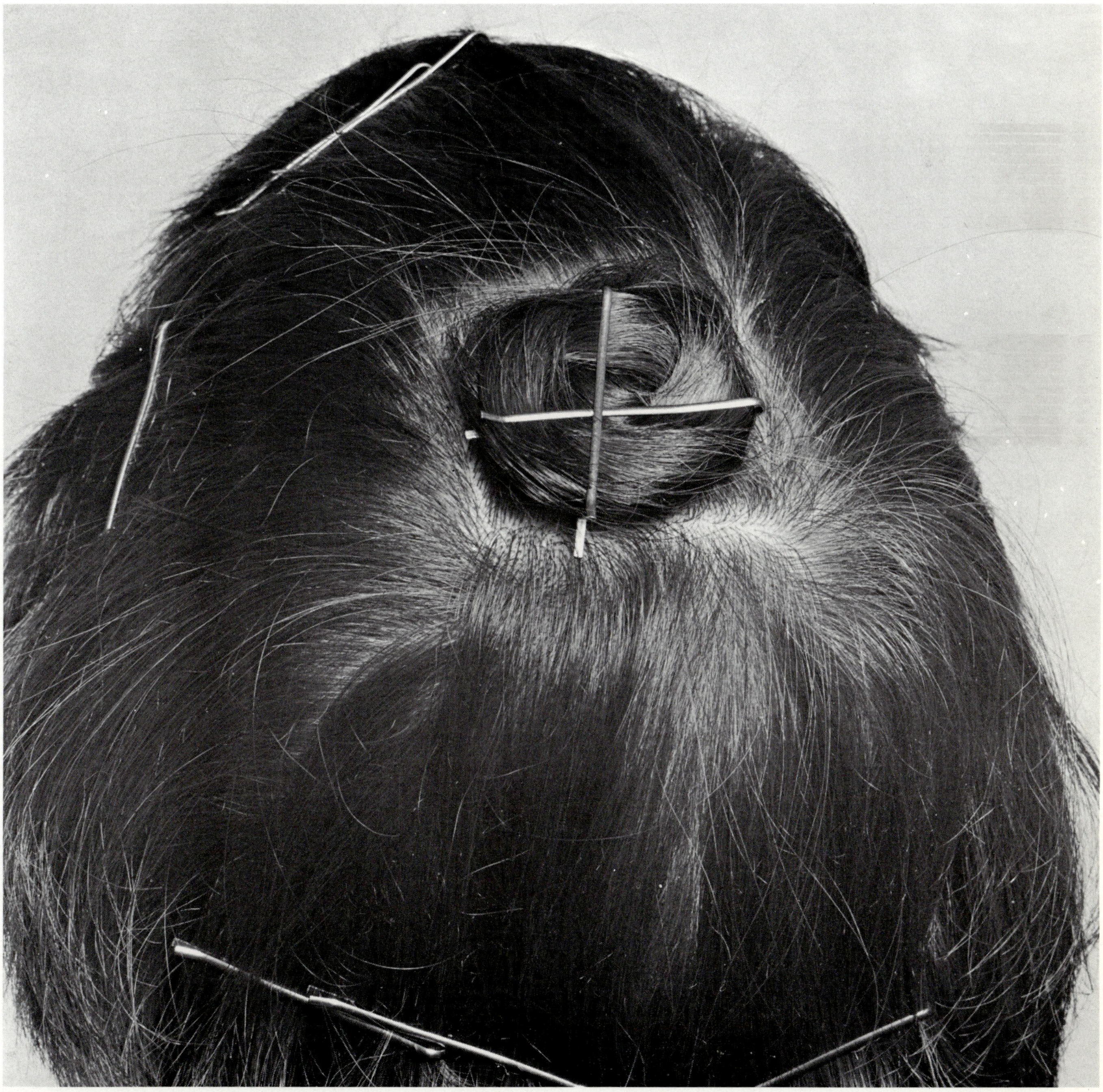

43 Then slip the fixing comb attached to the base well under the pincurl.

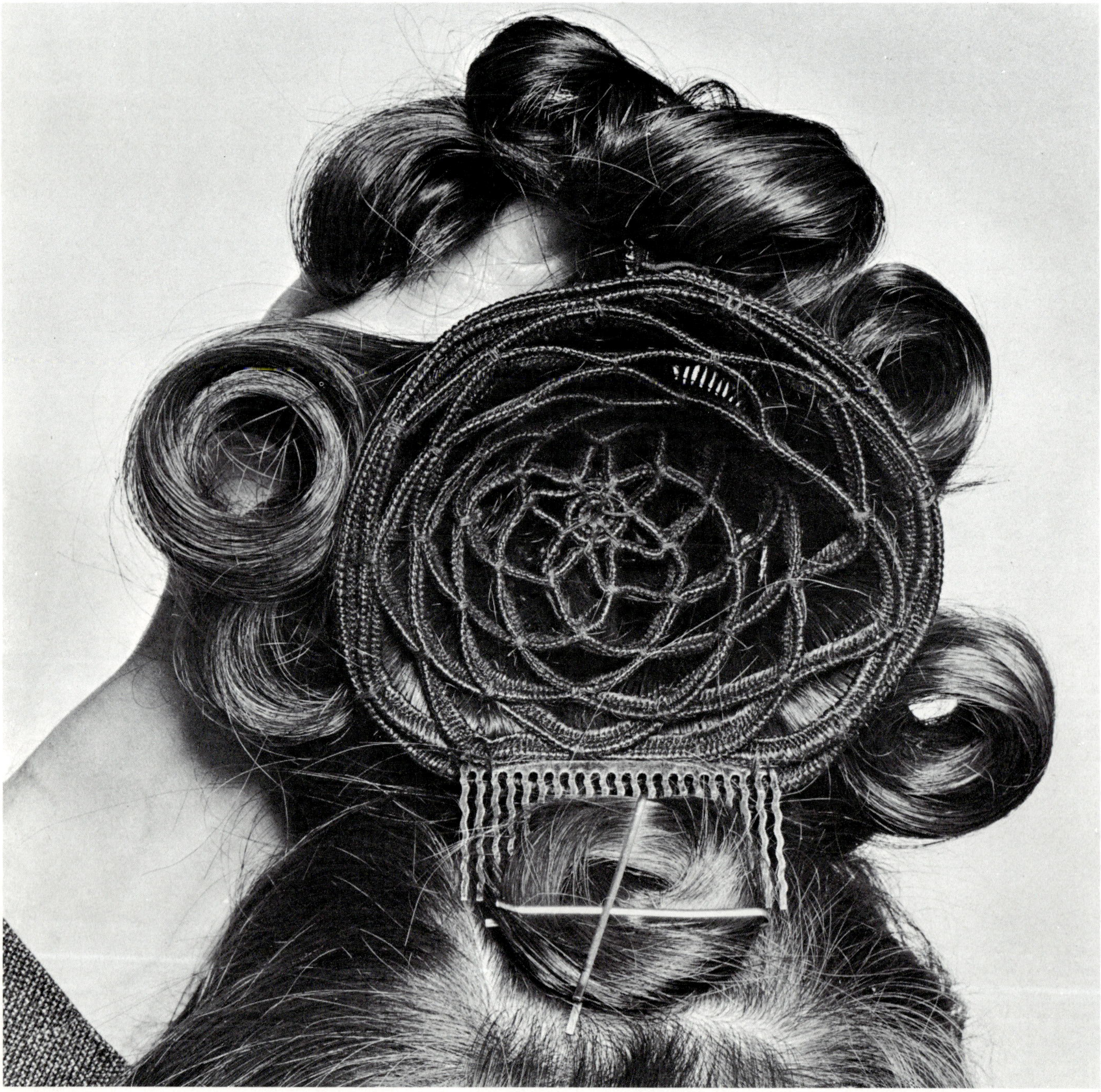

44 Next bring the base forward and over until it lies flat against the customer's head. Secure by half-inserting strong hairpins or grips at regular intervals round the rim of the base. Take care not to pierce the base fibres. Then push the hairgrips in fully. Finally give the hairpiece a tug to check that it is fixed really firmly.

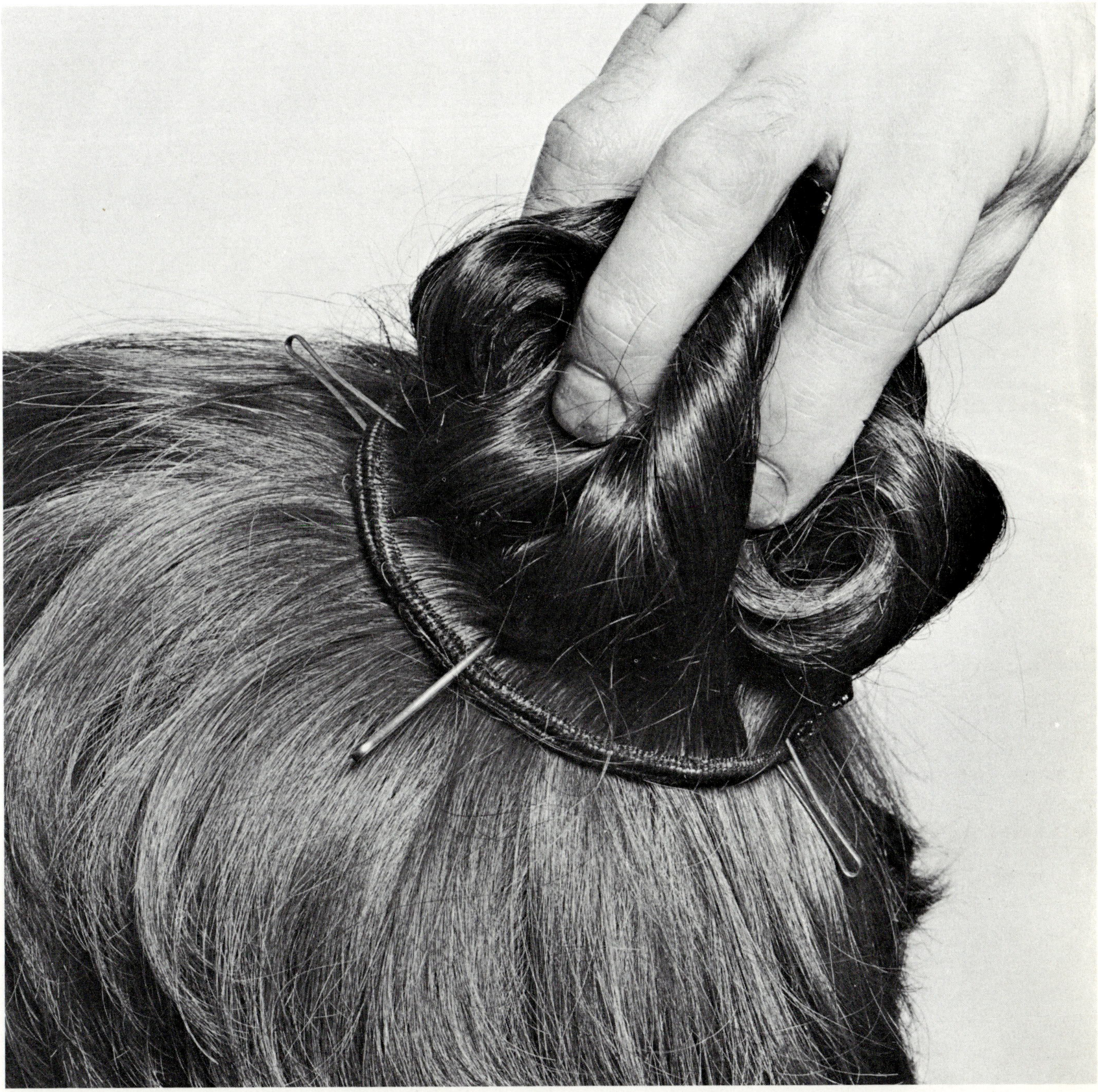

. . . and Putting on a Wig

First and most important—the customer's own hair must be pinned smoothly and firmly to her head. With slovenly pinning her hair can slip out beneath the edge of the wig later. Also lumpy pinning can spoil the whole shape of the wig.

A wig must always be put on front first. Place the centre point of the front in the middle of the customer's forehead. Ask her to hold it there. Then pull the wig well down into the back of her neck. Push the front back to the natural hairline making sure the ears are on the outside of the wig. Check round the hairline to see that none of the customer's hair is showing beneath and make sure she feels comfortable in the wig.

Alterations

Non-stretch foundations do loosen after a great deal of wear. When this happens, though, it is quite easy to reduce the slack and make it a perfect fit again. First fit the wig on the customer's head, making sure the centre front corresponds with the middle of her forehead. Then feel around the edge of the foundation to find out where it is loose. If it does not fit snugly behind the ears, as it should, darts must be made to remove excess bulk.

45 If the wig is too large over the ear sections, a dart should be made from behind the ear shaping *diagonally* towards the crown.

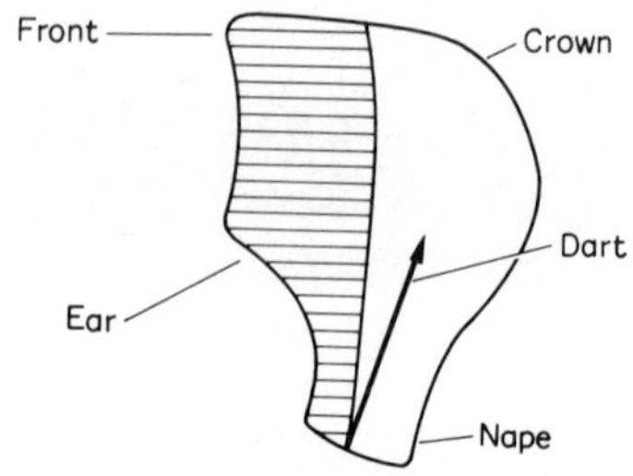

46 For larger alterations, another dart should be made in the centre nape section; this time *vertically* towards the crown. Mark the darts with pins to give an indication of the depth required.

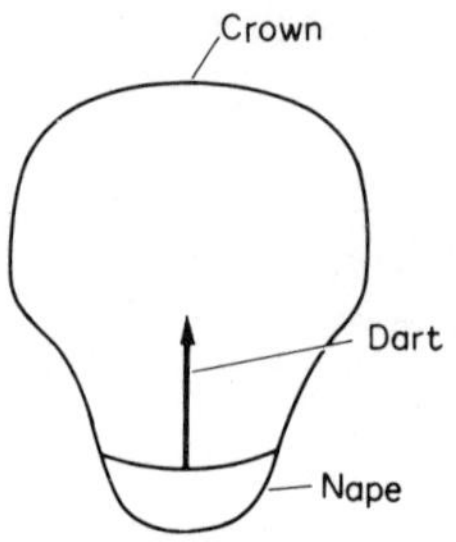

47 The wig should be turned inside out and the darts pinned in the direction of the diagrams on opposite page. The wig is then re-placed on the customer's head to check the fit.

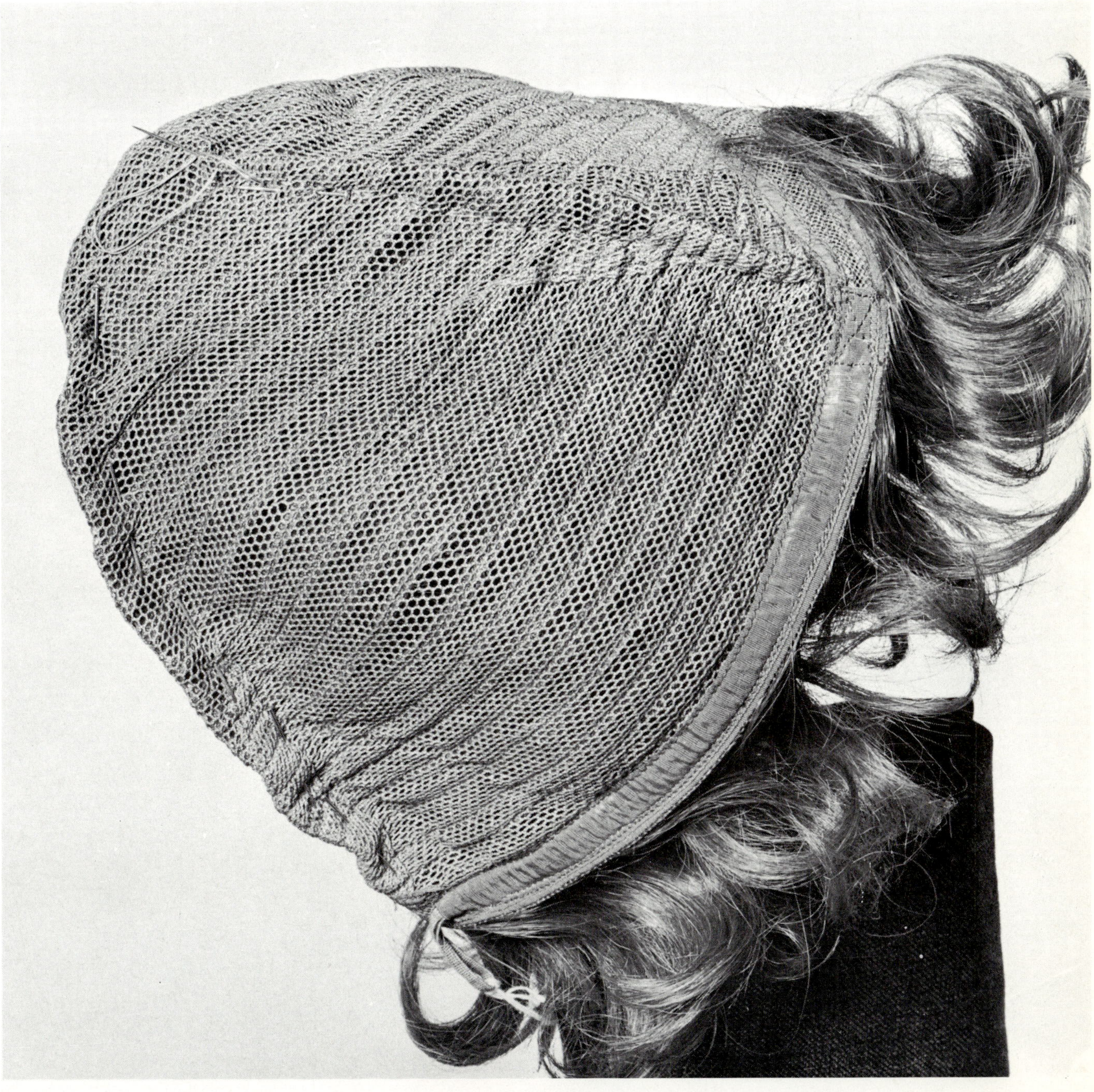

48 To make darts, back-stitch along the required depth of the dart, tapering at both ends as in the diagram, Figure 49.

49

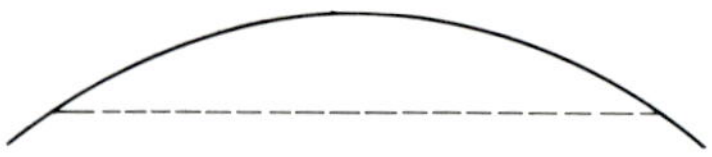

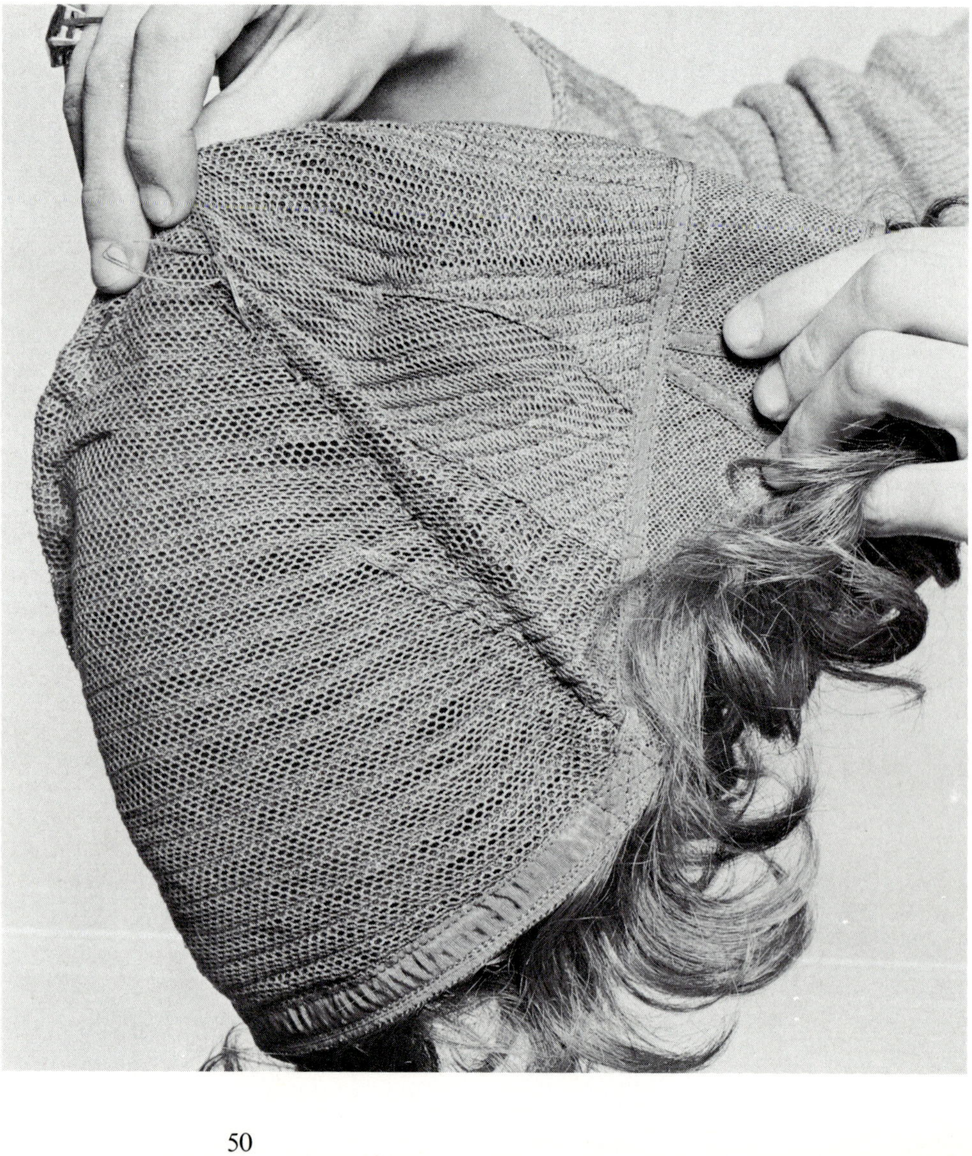

50 Next press each dart down towards the centre so that it lies flat against the foundation. Oversew along the loose edge.

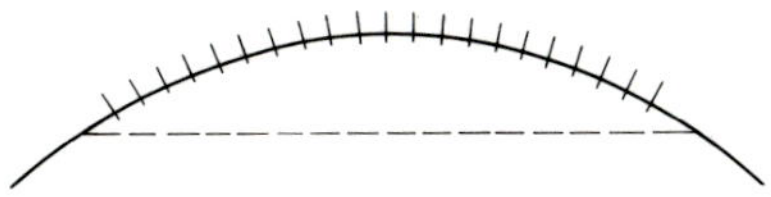

51 The finished dart with all bulk flattened out giving a neater fit.

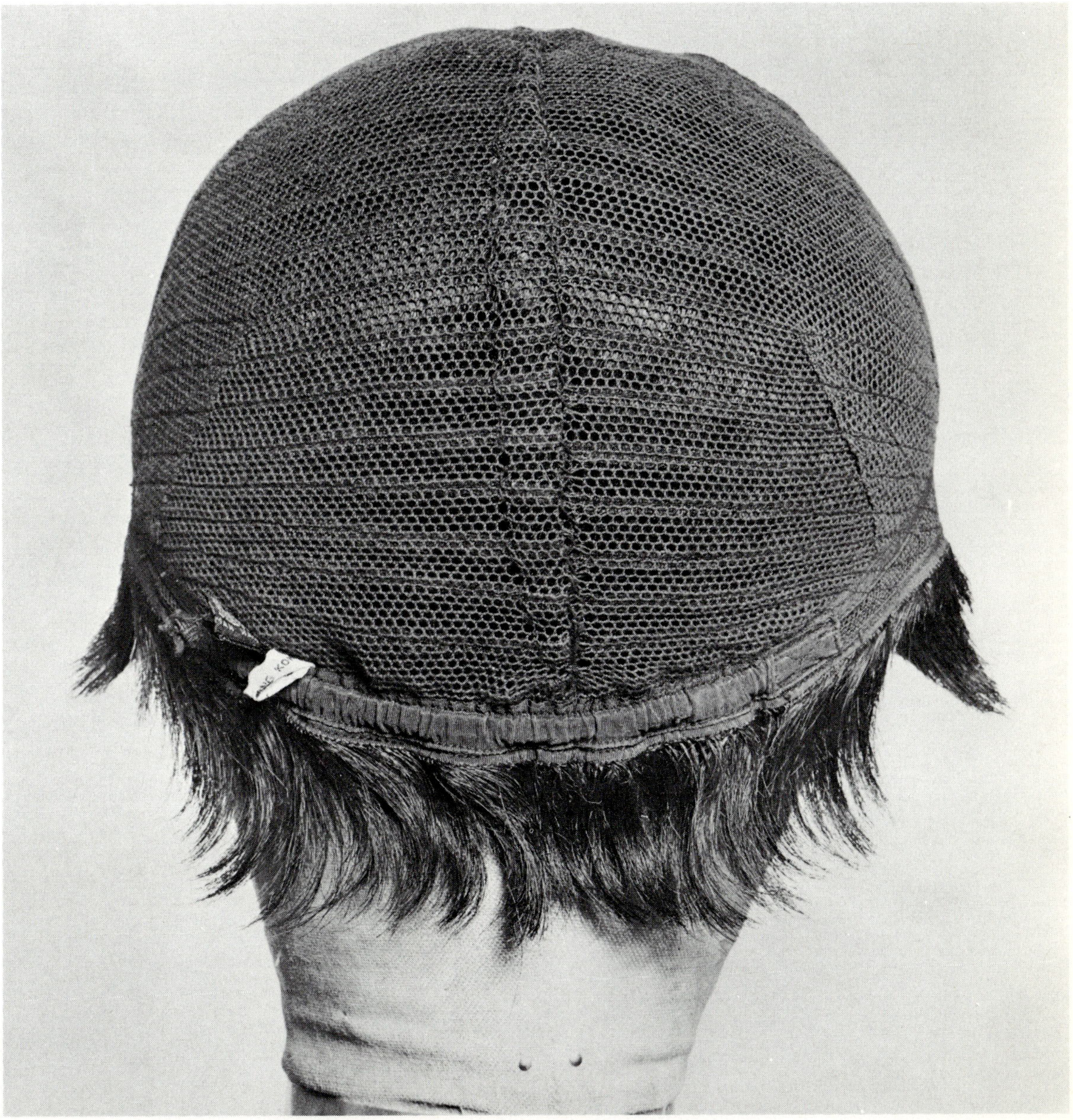

Professional Presentation

The superfine taper-cut

A really well-cut wig is a natural looking one. The hair is finely shaped and fits snugly round the face and neck. Ruthless tapering to eliminate hair bulk is the secret. Here, provided you are an expert at cutting, is a demonstration of the razor-cutting technique on Asian hair.

Before you begin, determine the length of hair for any style at three points: nape, centre, and over each of the ears. Remember that hair wigs should be cut *wet*, with a razor, and fibre ones *dry*, with thinning scissors.

52 It's hard to believe this is a wig. It is, though, an Asian hair one. This is what superfine razoring can do to create a completely natural look.

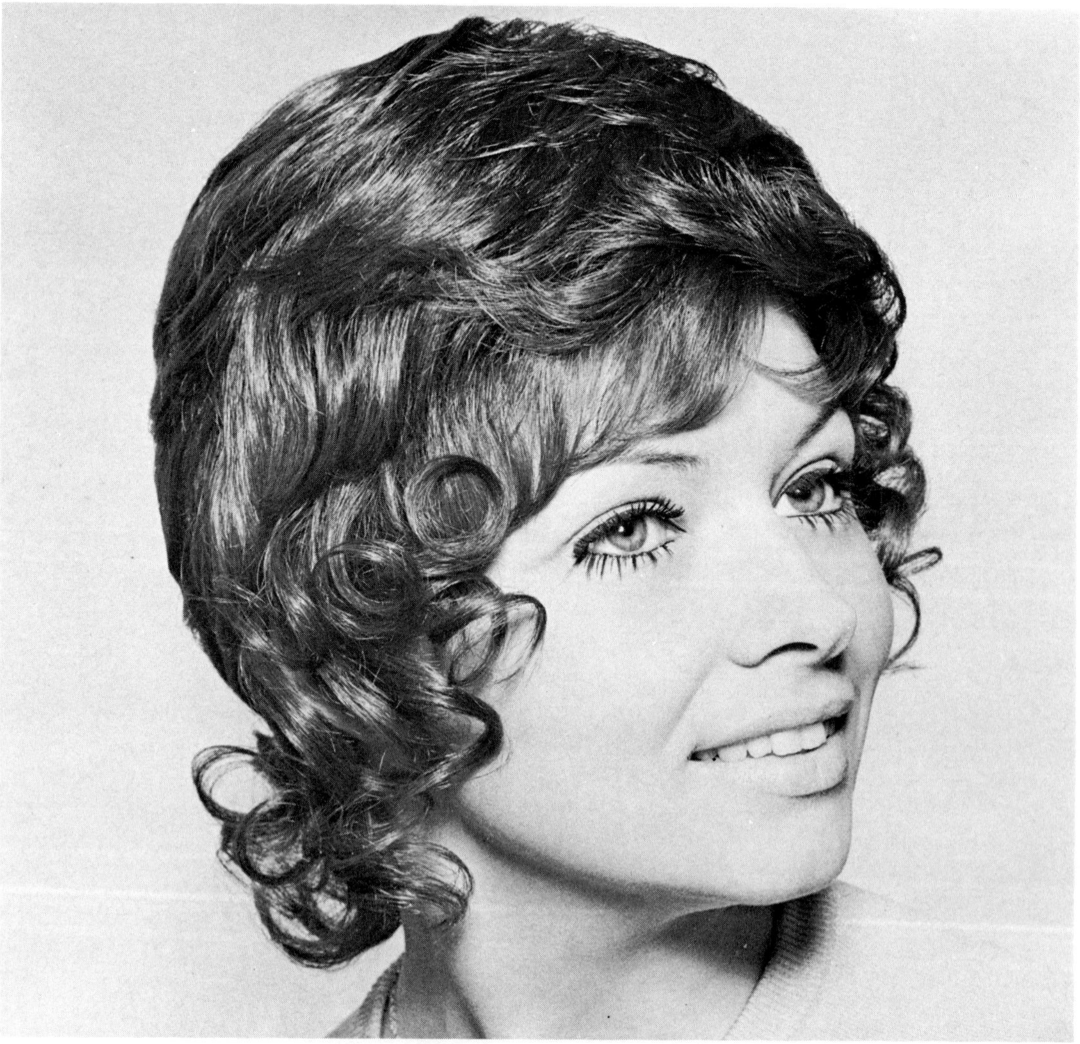

53 The uncut wig, correctly blocked, and with the hair thoroughly dampened, ready for razor cutting. The basic cutting shape of the design is a layered cap, a side fringe, and long side and nape hair.

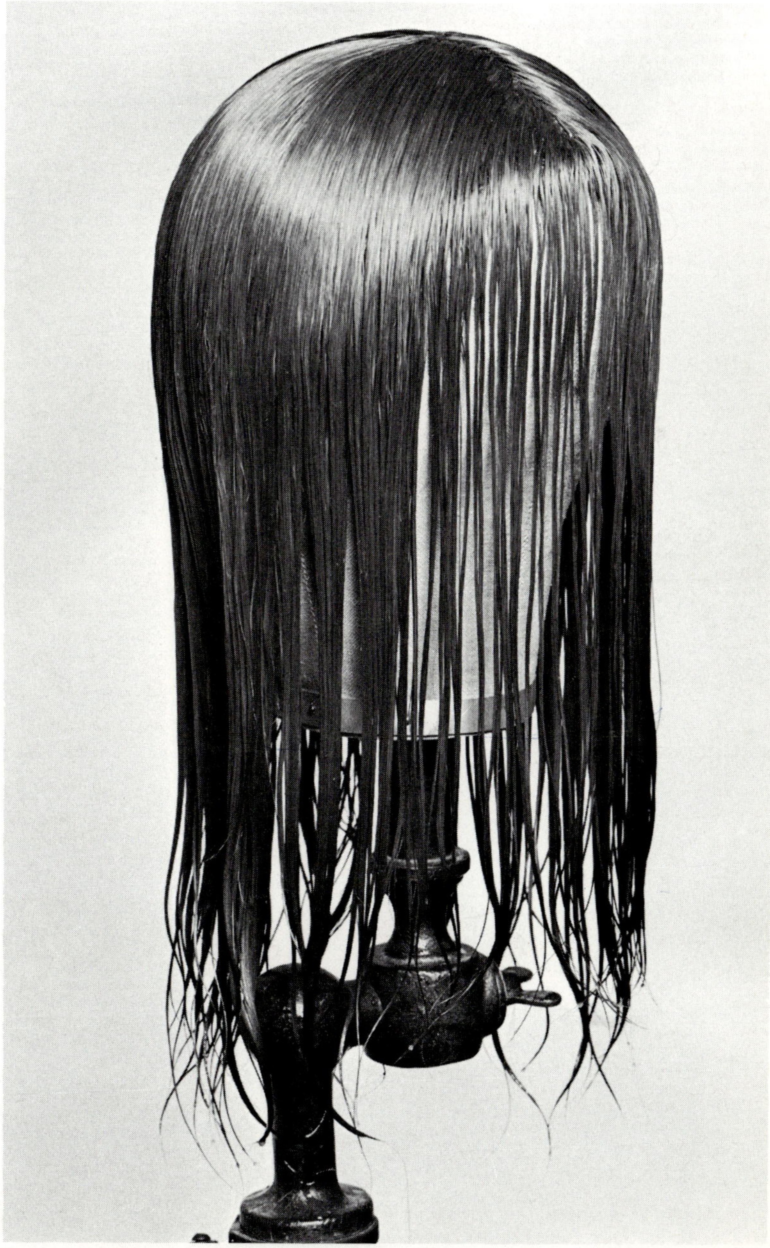

54 First comes fine sectioning of the hairline where the hair is thickest. The rest of the hair is pinned into a cap-shape out of the way.

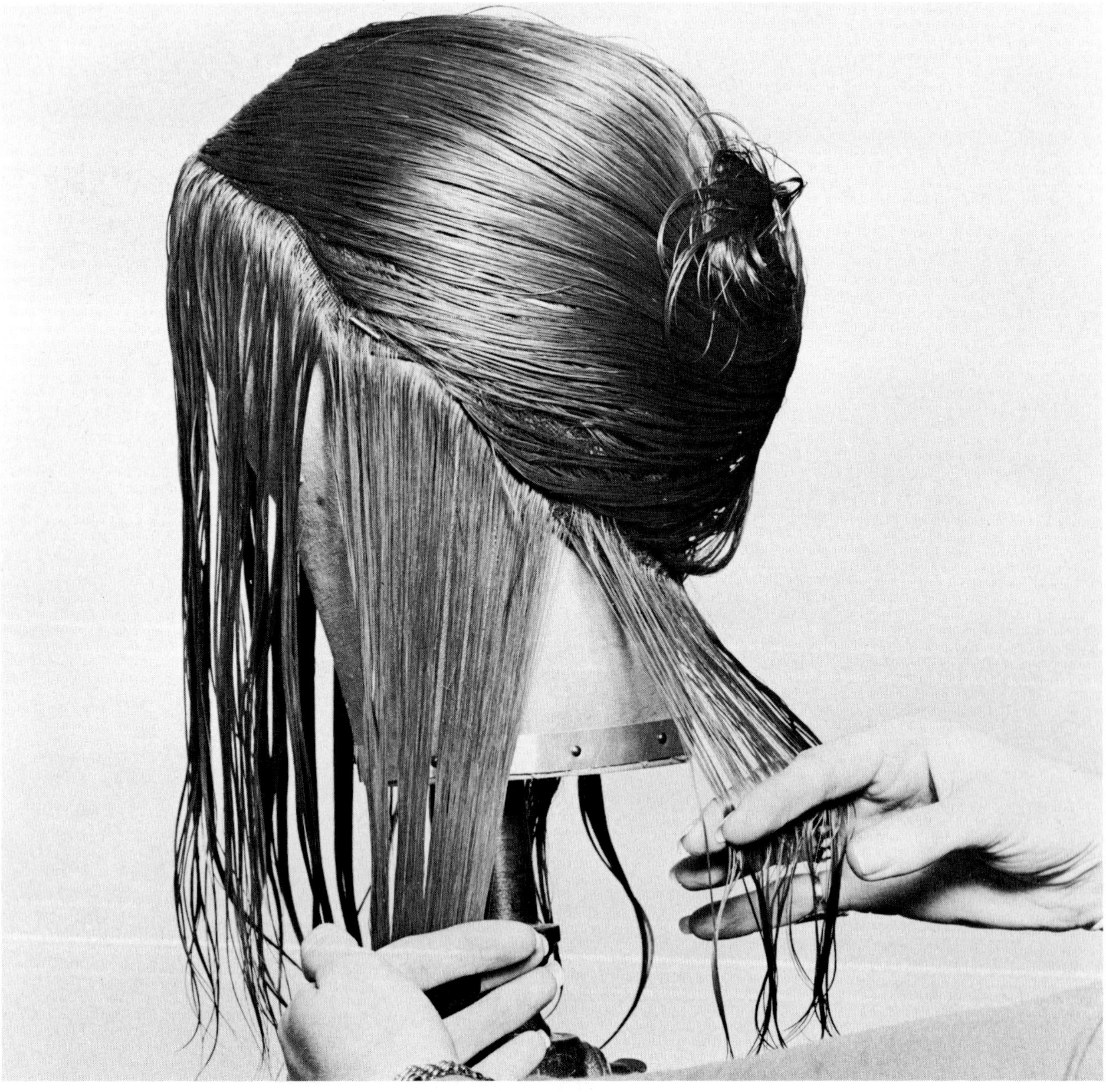

55 The hairline section is then razor cut, working to within 3 cm (1 in.) of the roots. This is the degree of thinning required for a close-fitting hairline.

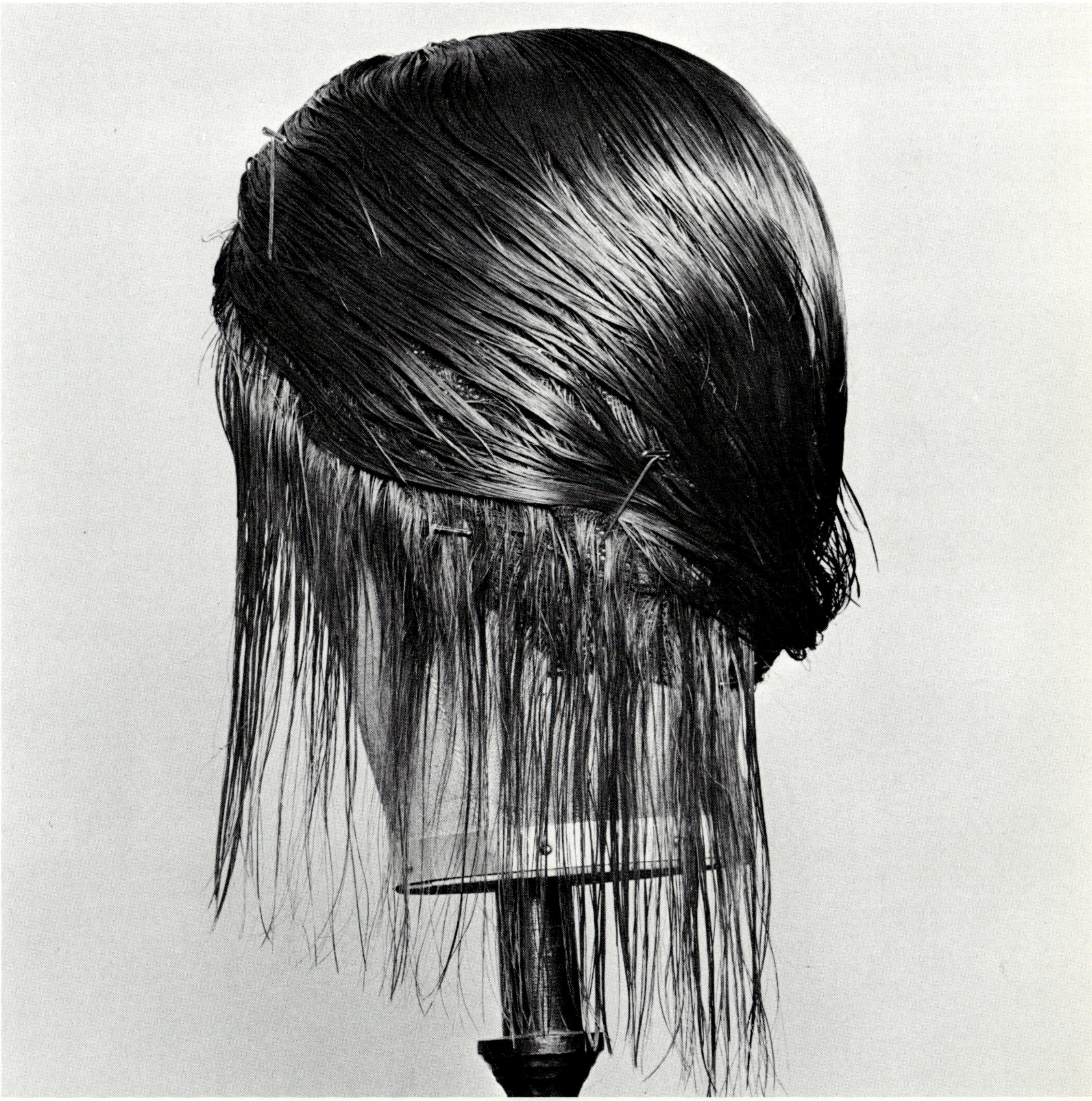

56 Razoring the fringe—another part which needs drastic thinning to avoid an over-heavy look.

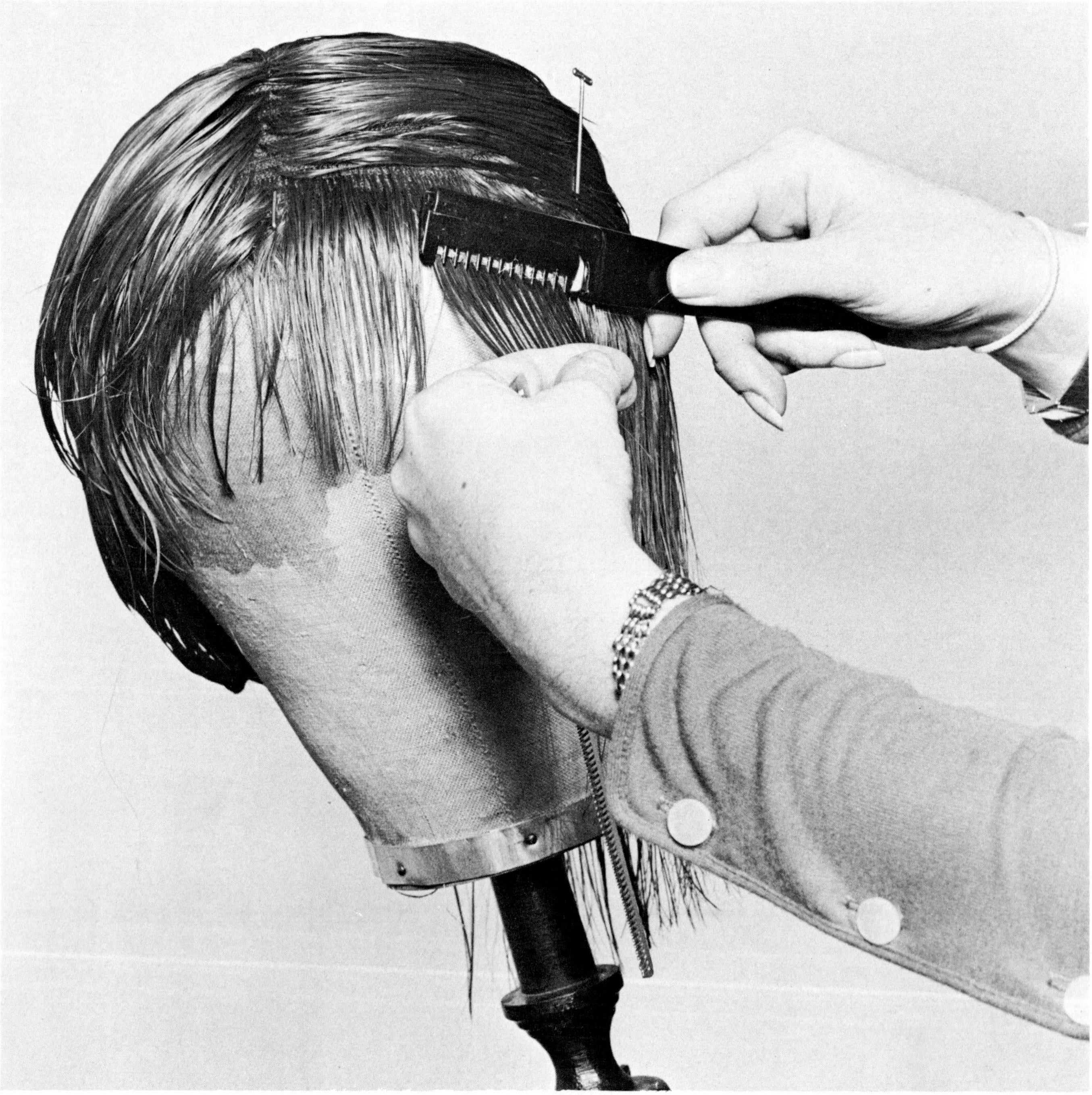

57 A wide tissue strip pinned below the cap shape helps to show up the hair and acts as a guide for future layering.

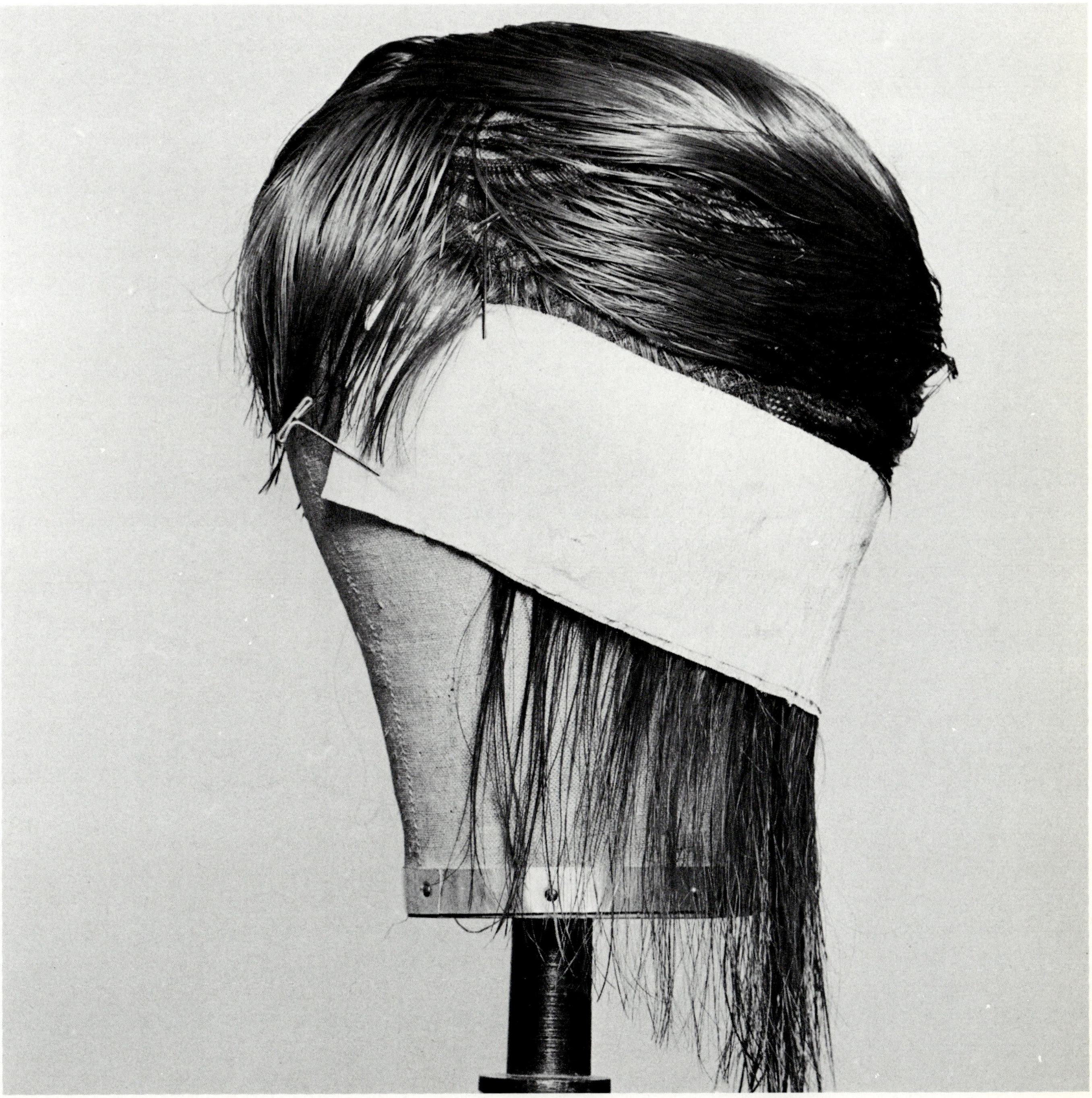

58 Now comes layering the hair within the cap-shape. The bottom layer is the first to be tackled, one side at a time.

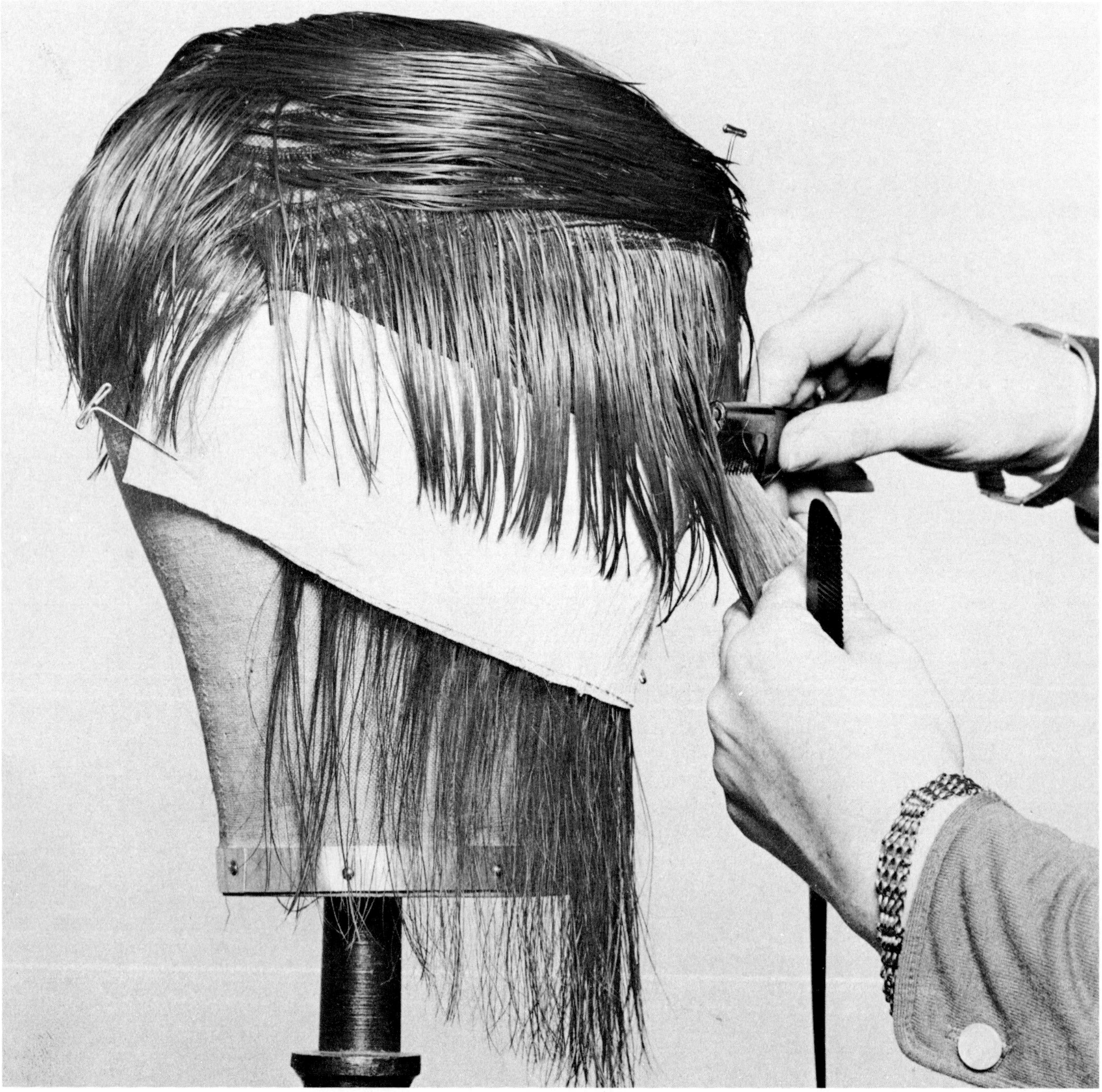

59 A comb-through next to check length and direction.

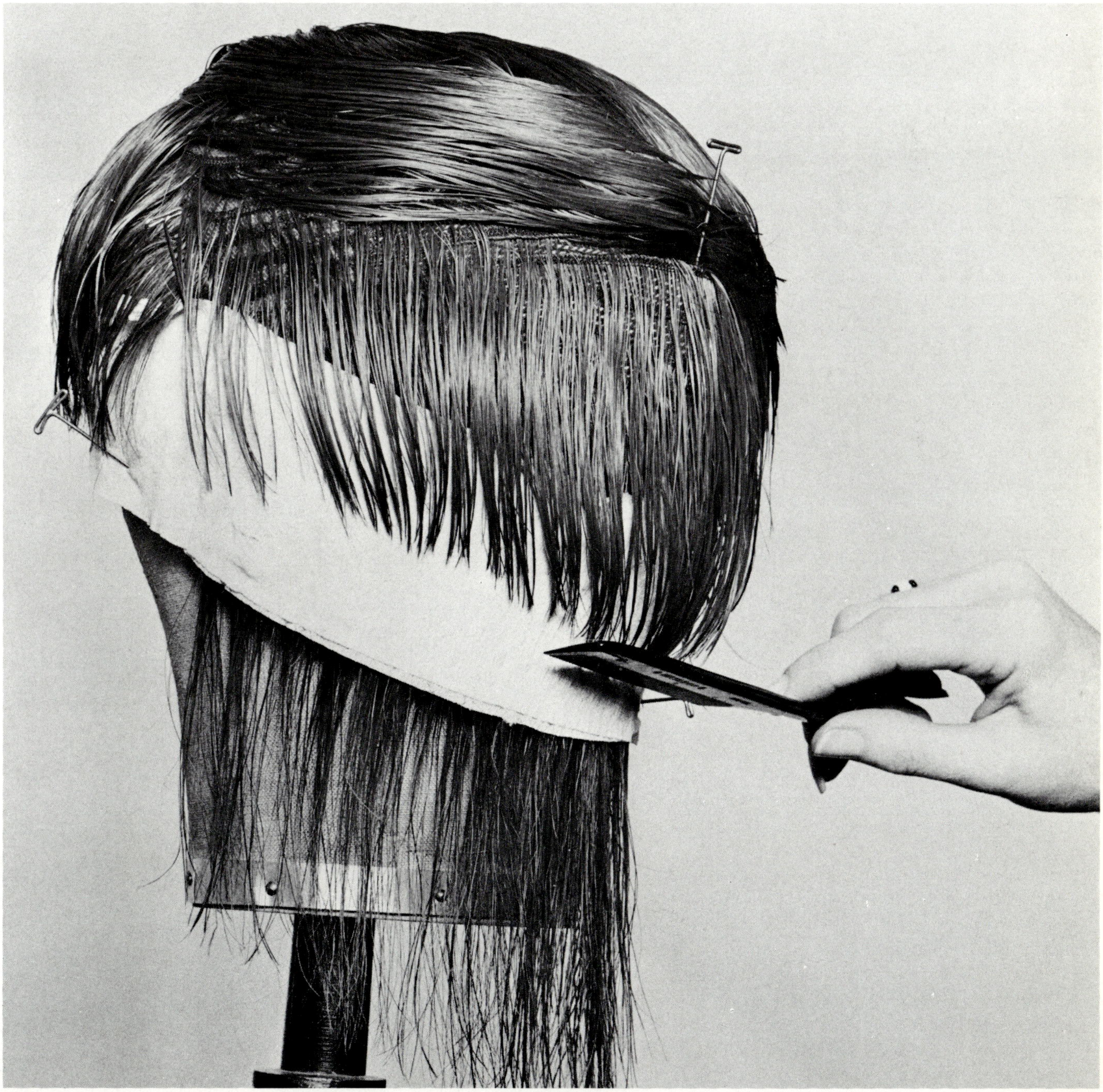

60 Layering is continued, working upwards towards the crown.

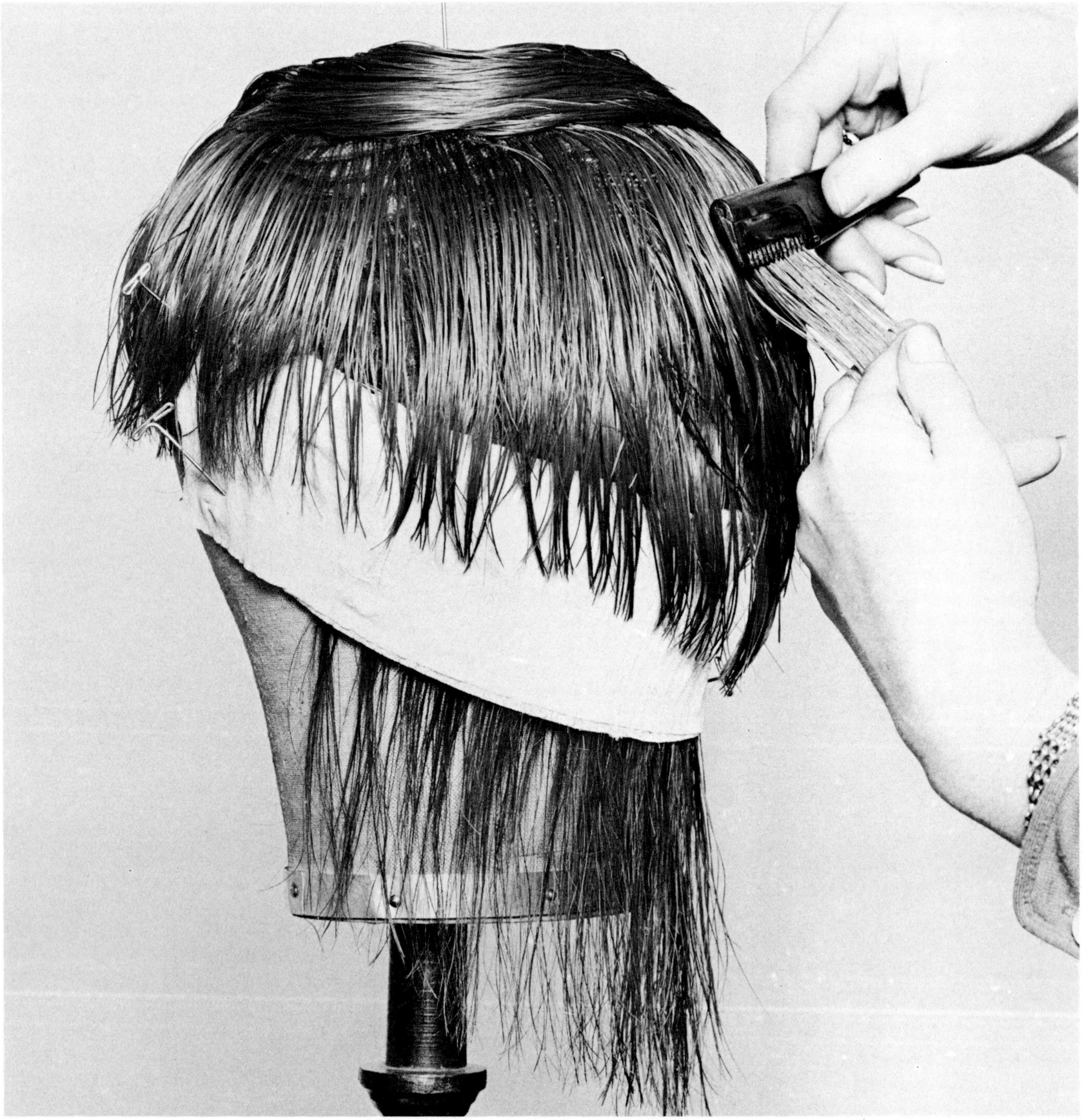

61 The crown hair needs less thinning than any of the hair, so layers are taken only to within 3 centimetres (1 inch) of it.

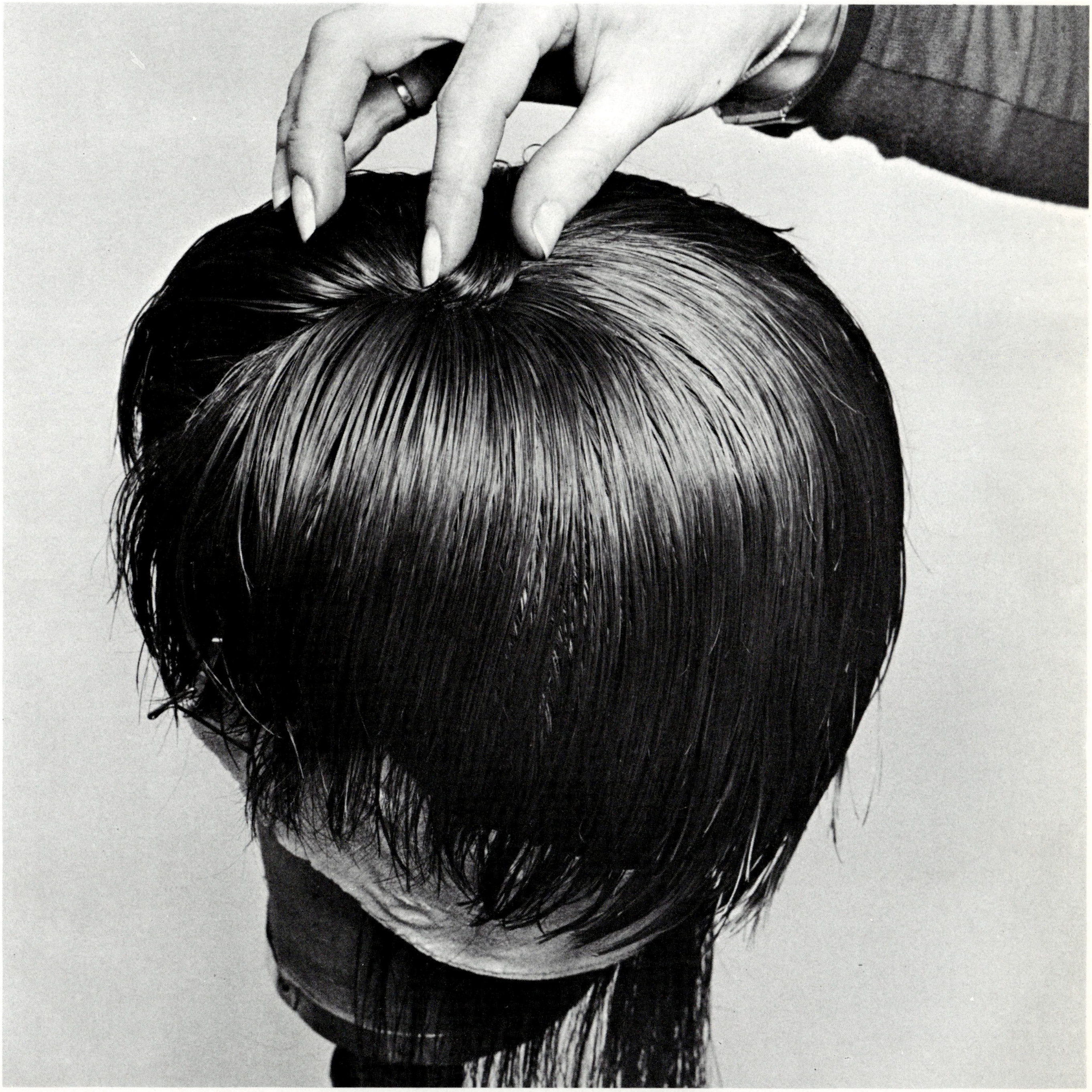

62 A check with scissors to see that layers correspond with each other, and a levelling off of any ragged ends.

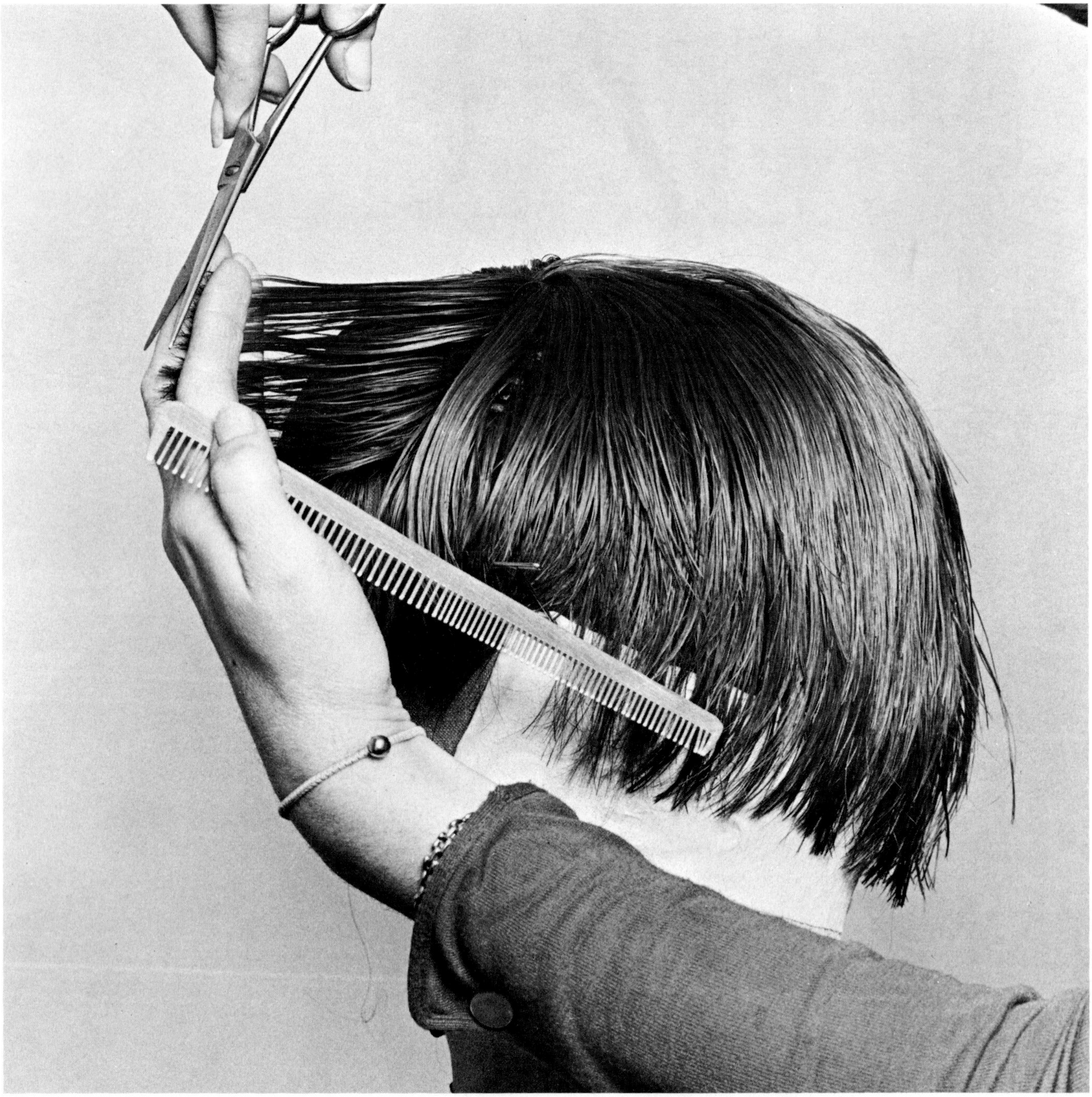

63 The finished cut—superb shaping with all layers blending in with each other. Note the complete absence of bulk anywhere.

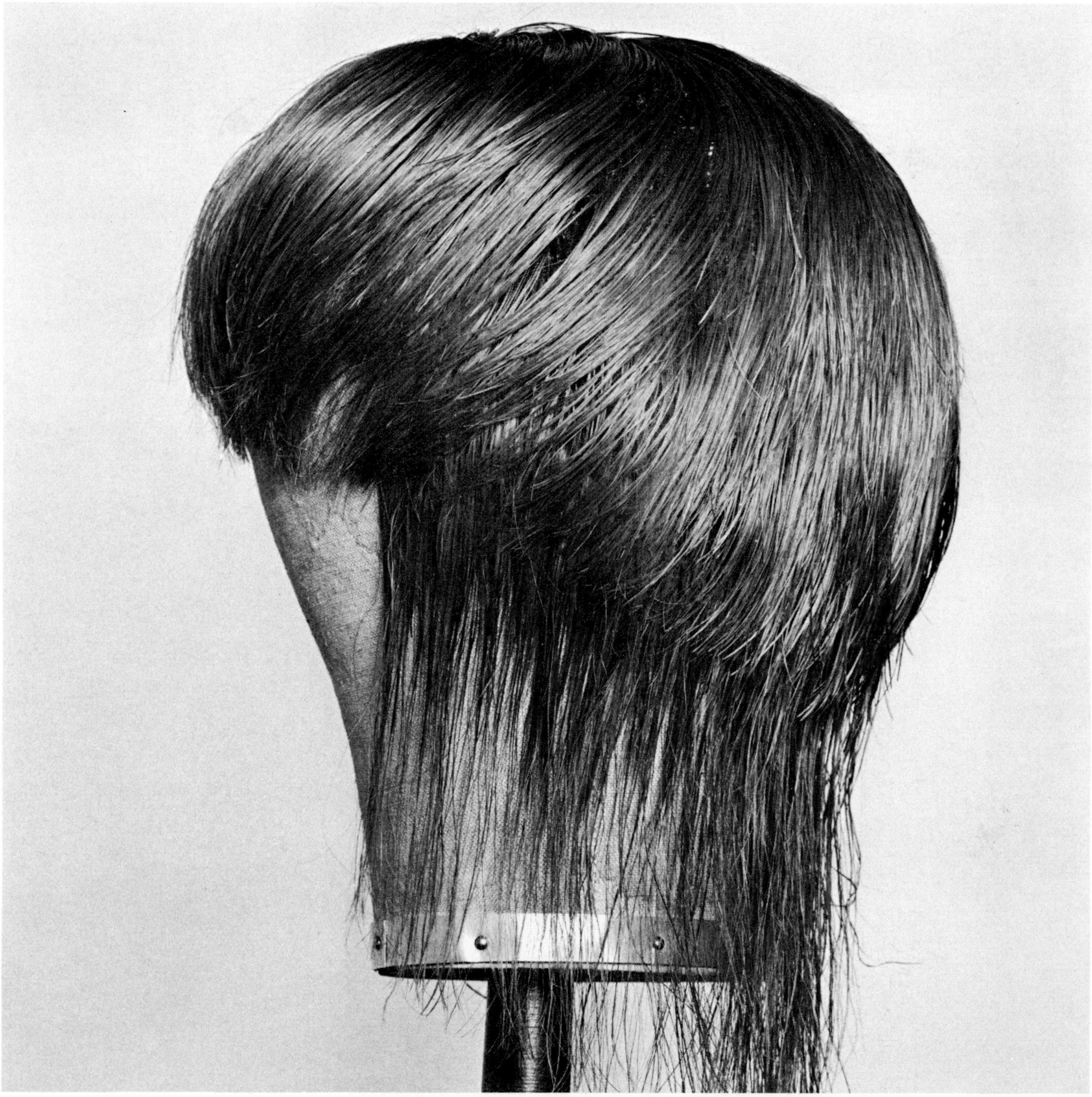

64 A prominent crown must be disguised by rollering around the point.

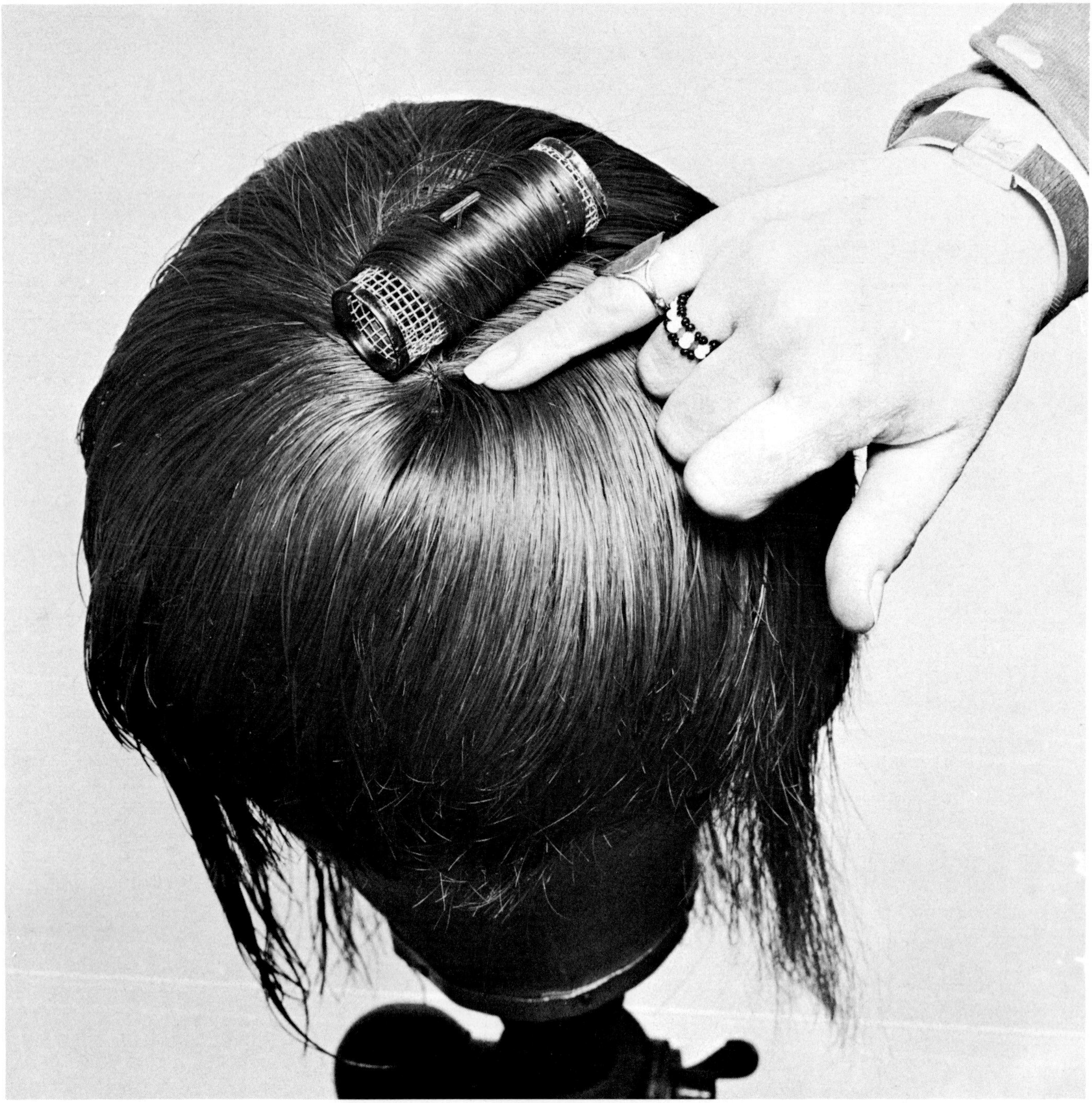

. . . and the setting technique

65 The setting pattern or pli. The top hair layers are wound *under* on to smooth metal rollers. These should be staggered to avoid gaps at comb-out. Placement should follow the forward movement of the hair and the direction of the fringe. Side hair is wound on curlers *towards* the face. The rest of the hair and fringe is moulded into shape and anchored with T-pins. Then the wig is put under a hot hair-dryer for four hours to dry out. When the hair is unwound it must be left to cool before comb-out.

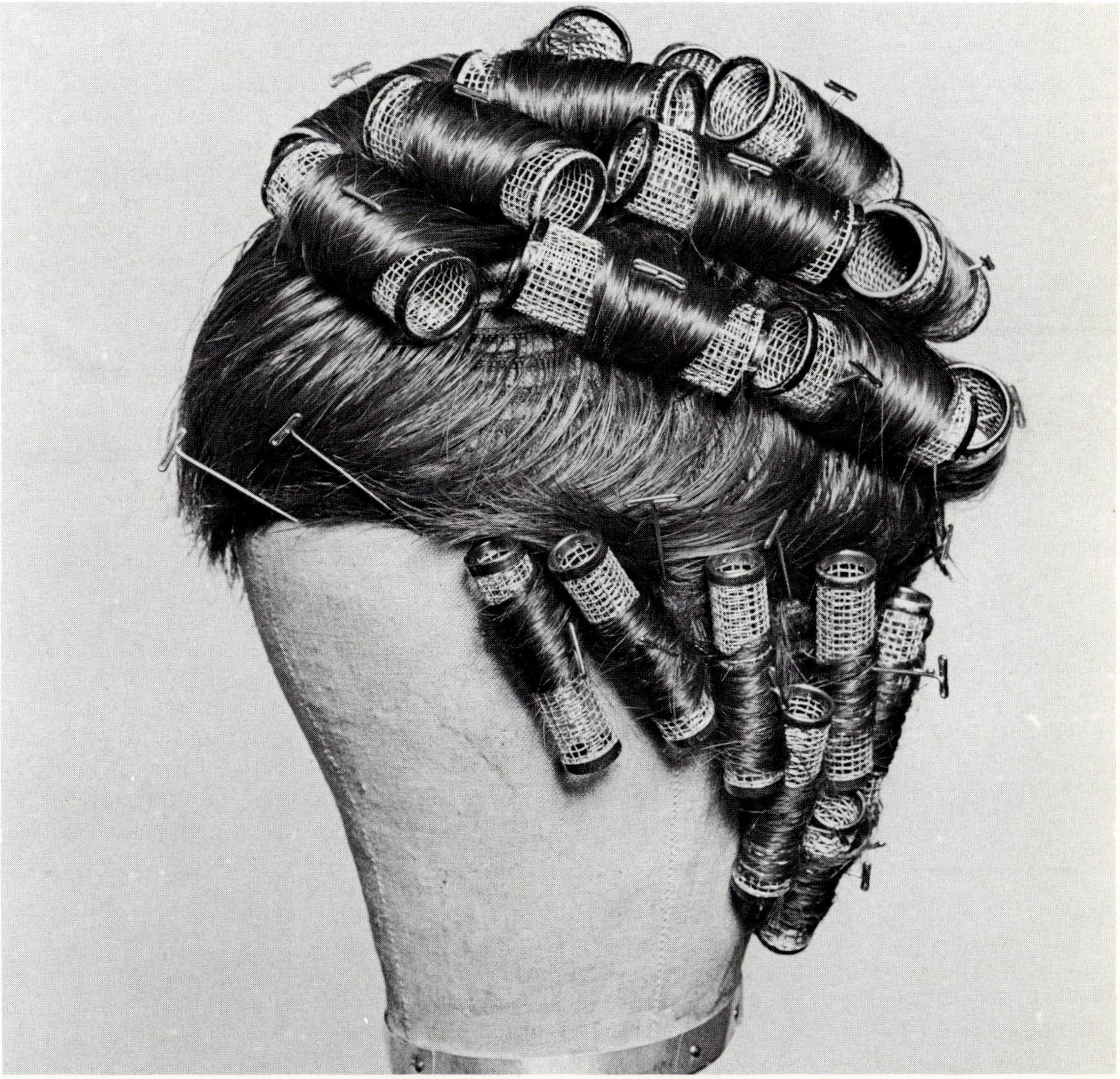

66 When the hair is unwound, any separation marks between rollers can be removed with a hand-dryer at a hot setting.

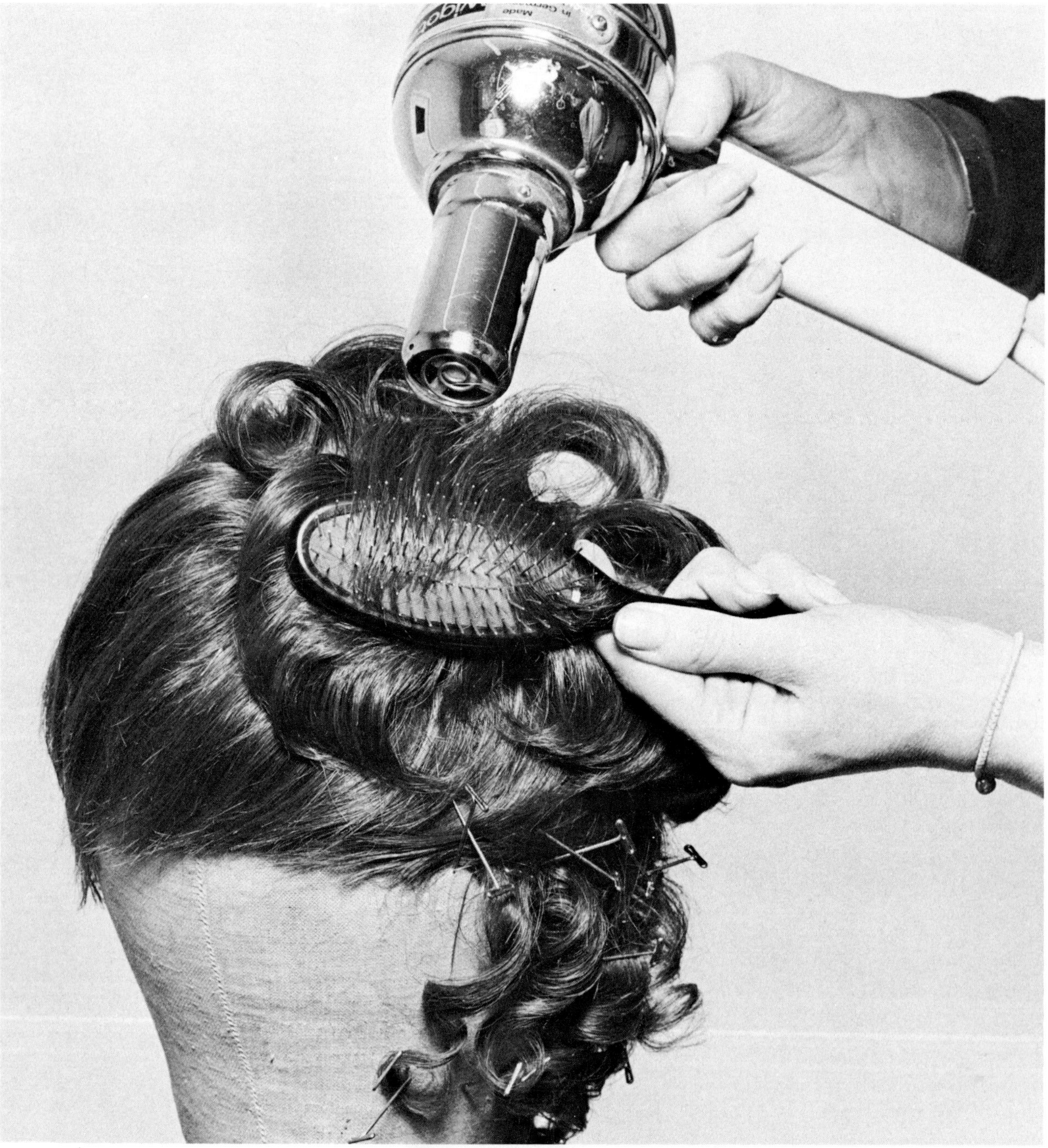

67 To give the style its curving movement, unwound hair is lifted away from the foundation with electric curling tongs to form a series of half-curls.

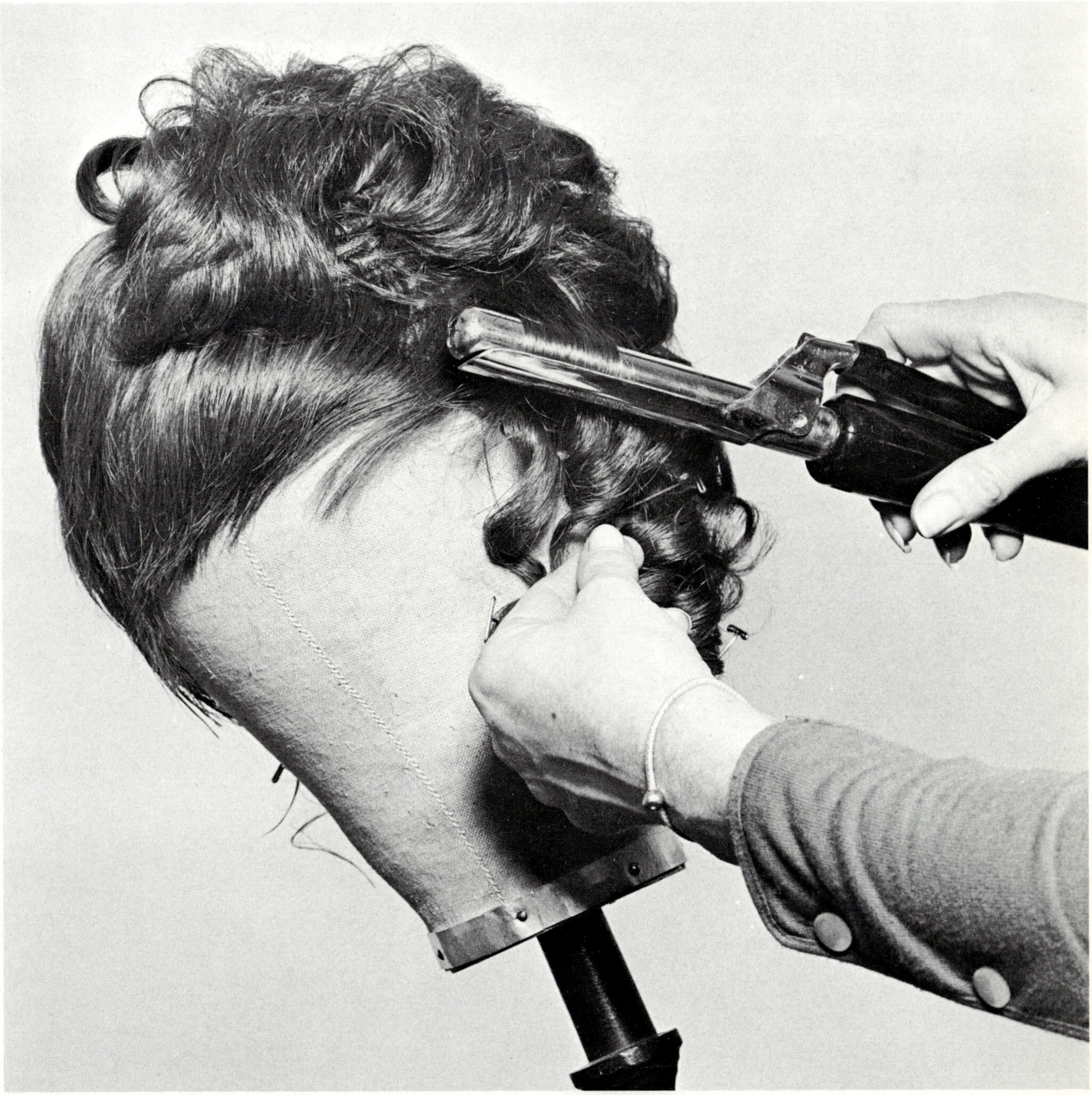

Cutting to the face

A wig taken out of its plastic bag and brushed into shape on the customer's head is not the best way to make a sale. A more personalized approach will have greater success, particularly with the older women. Although most fibre wigs are pre-cut and ready-to-wear, they can be improved by professional attention. Thinning and trimming uneven ends plus back-brushing and re-styling, to suit individual features, should be part of customer presentation. Any upgrading of the general image of wigs can lead to better business.

68 Out of the bag and on to the head—a long curly fibre wig designed for the young. All a girl needs to do is brush it into shape.

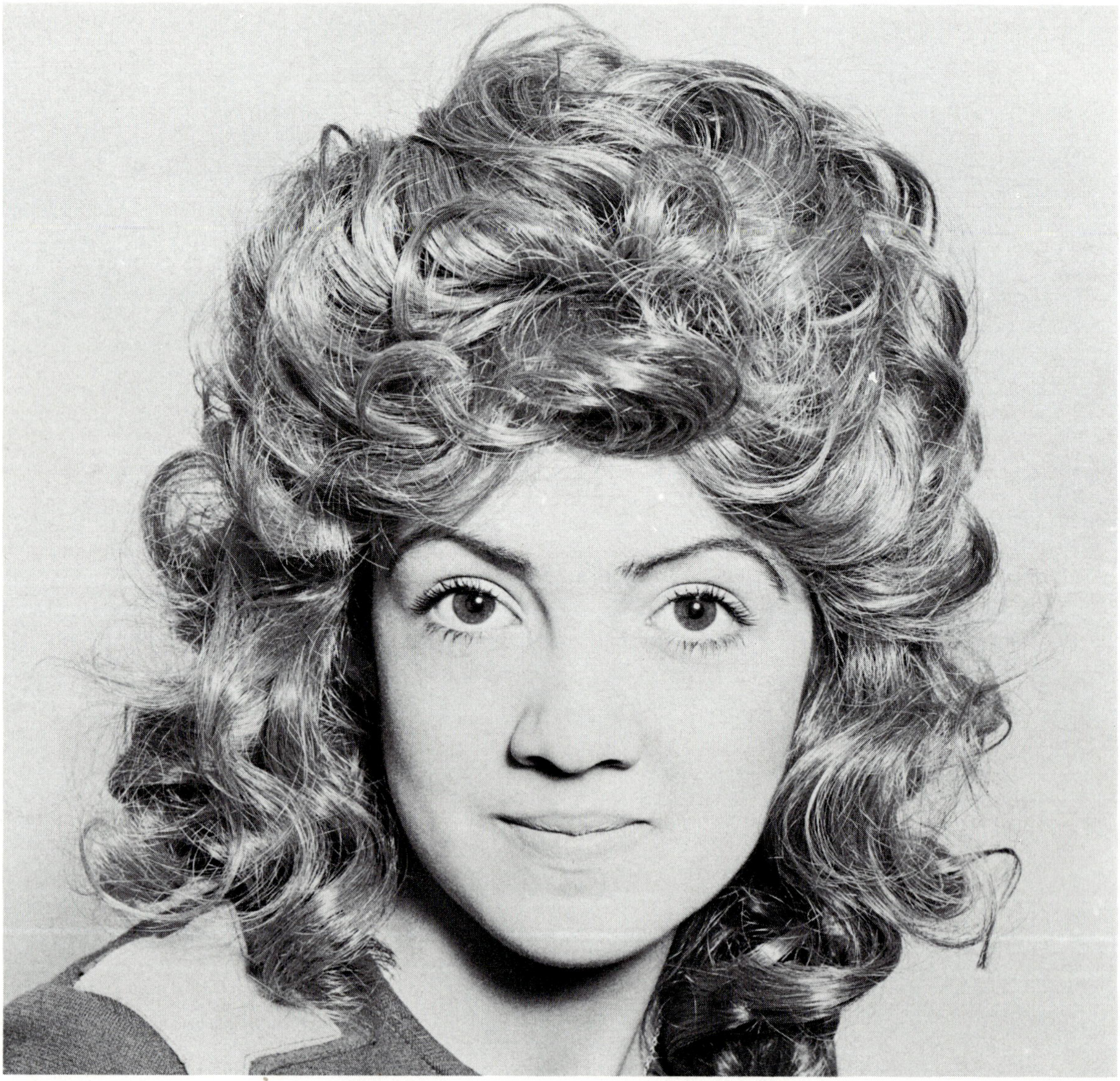

69 The same wig with a more professional look preferred by a lot of women. The ends have been trimmed with thinning scissors and the hair backbrushed and re-styled.

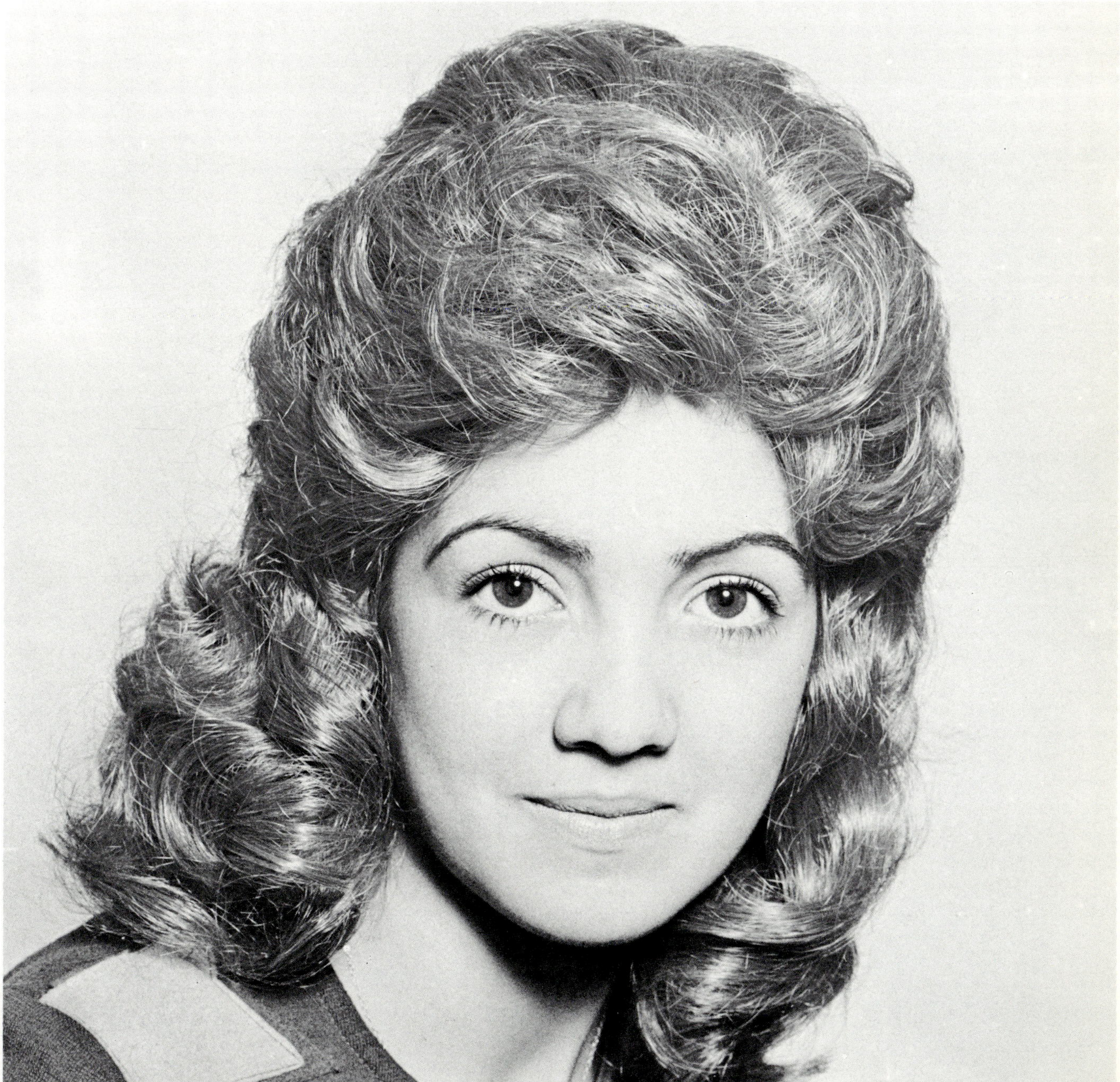

70 Creating an entirely different effect with the same wig. The front is cut and tapered to suit the face while the wig is on the customer's head.

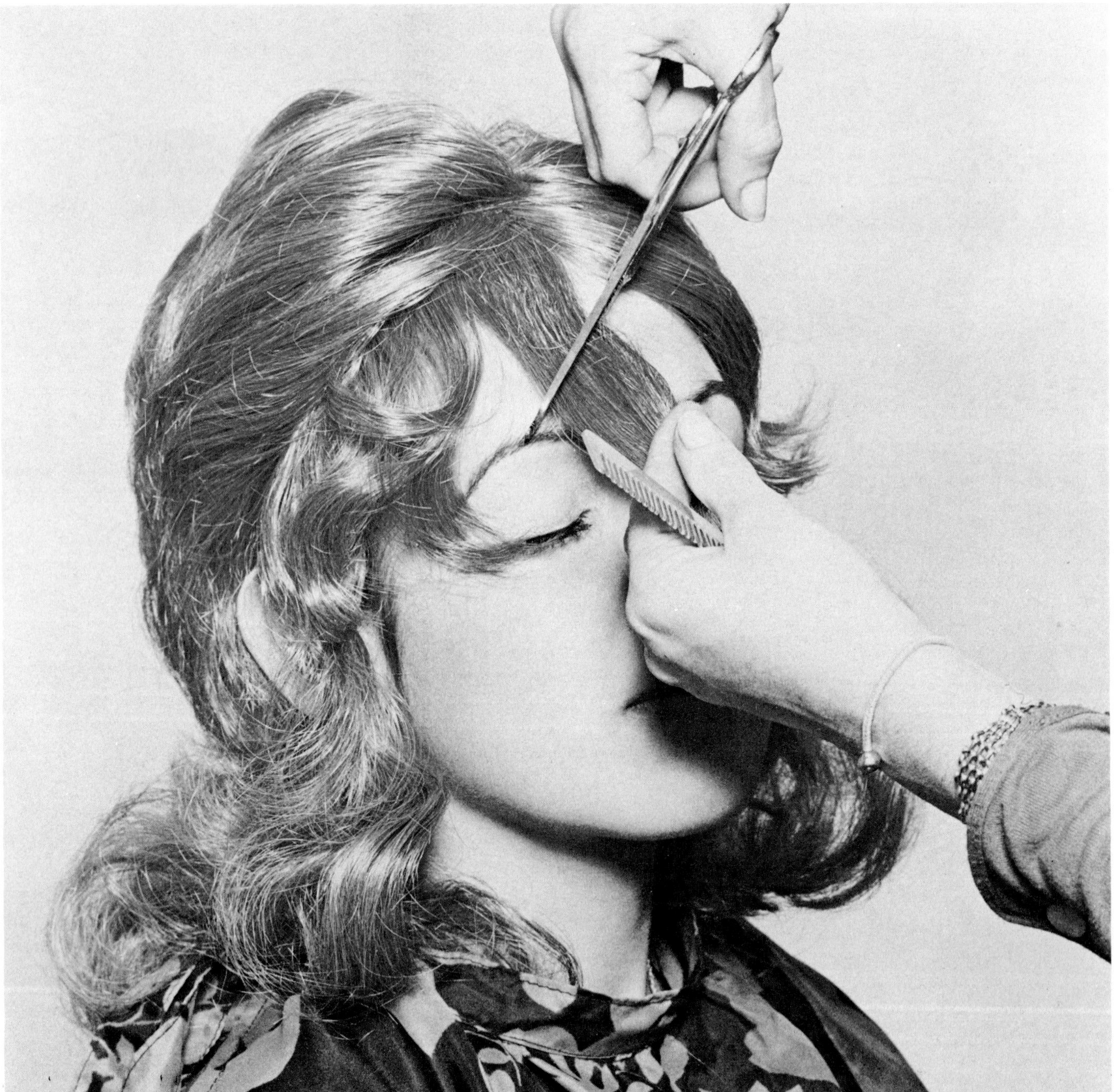

71 Then the top layers are brushed smoother and long curving sidepieces brought forward over the ears.

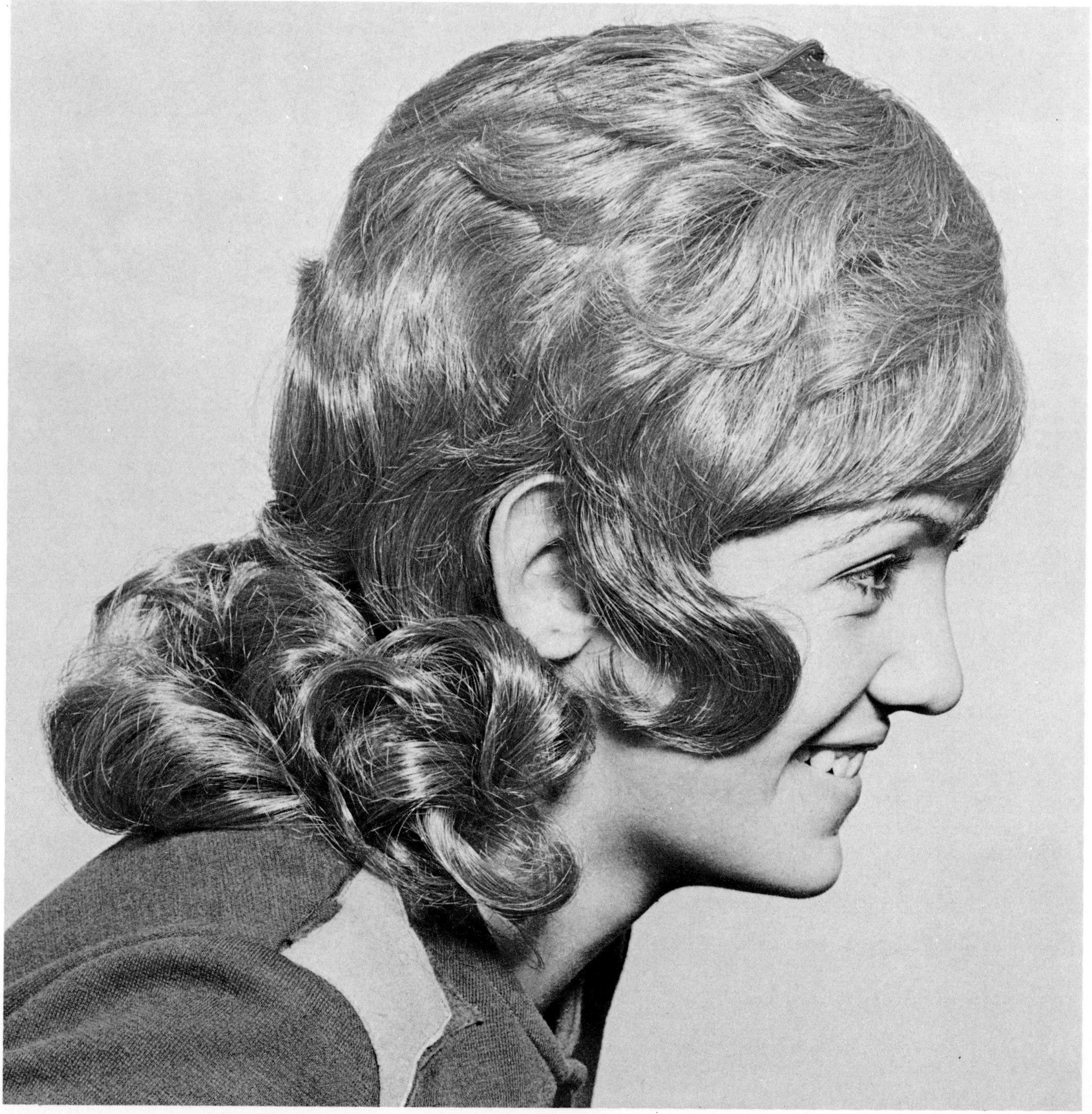

Cleaning and Conditioning Hair

No two people agree on the best cleaning methods for Asian hair. Some believe in spraying on the cleaner and combing it thoroughly through the hair. Not enough, say others who advocate gentle agitation in cleaning solution. Then there is another school which insists on shaking the wig in a screw-topped jar filled with cleaning fluid. On the other hand, there are the purists who maintain that shampooing is the only way to remove every particle of grease and dirt. So there are no hard and fast rules for beginners. It all depends on the following conditions:

1. The quality and category of hair, and the type of base or foundation.
2. The degree of regularity with which the wig or hairpiece is worn.
3. The amount of excess grease produced by the wearer's scalp. This varies from woman to woman.

There is one golden rule, however, when it comes to shampooing. Never even contemplate washing unless the wig or hairpiece is clearly labelled washable or you are able to check back with the supplier. Whichever cleaning method you choose, though, remember these important points.

a. Always protect the foundation from damage or distortion.

b. Wherever possible, do not try to speed up the drying process. Try to allow the hair to dry out naturally, well away from any kind of heater or radiator.

c. Above all, clean wigs and hairpieces at regular intervals. Never allow them to become over-soiled. If you do, like natural hair, the wig will quickly become limp and lustreless and all that much harder to restore to its initial gloss and bounce.

The dry-clean method

The Solutions . . .

Some real hair wigs or hairpieces can be washed. Others cannot. However, they can all be dry-cleaned with a special wig cleaner, which will remove a normal amount of dirt and grease successfully. Most modern wig cleaners are safe to use in confined spaces. A few are not, though—those containing carbon tetrachloride. Although non-inflammable and a first-class de-greaser, it gives off fumes which could be dangerous if used without sufficient ventilation.

Another type of wig cleaner contains trichlorethylene, a grease solvent. This, too, is non-inflammable but it also gives off dangerous fumes. Again, it must be used only where there is plenty of ventilation. Benzine is considered the most efficient cleaner by some wig specialists. But, of course, it is highly inflammable and gives off very dangerous fumes. It must, therefore, always be used out of doors, well away from any naked flames. Also it has special storage regulations which make it impractical for the average user.

. . . and the Way to Use Them

First make sure you have as much ventilation as possible in the room where you will be doing the cleaning. Make sure there are no naked flames or lighted cigarettes in the near vicinity. Hackle or brush the hair thoroughly first until all tangles have been removed. Place the piece or wig on a clean towel and spread out the hair. Or pin it firmly to a block.

Hold the aerosol cleaner can 15 to 25 cm (5–9 in.) away from the hair. Spray on the hair liberally, taking a small section at a time. Keep combing the cleaner through each section continuously. Repeat until all the hair is saturated and free from grease and dirt. Then thread fine wire through the base and hang the piece or wig up to dry naturally. When completely dried out, brush the hair thoroughly once again.

Deep-clean washing

Real hair wigs or hairpieces can be washed with several products—a special solution, wig washes or a mild shampoo. The same basic techniques apply and in this demonstration the special solution was used.

First all tangles are removed from the hair with hackle, brush or comb. Sufficient solution to cover the

72 Hackle—a flat board with upstanding metal teeth. Used for removing tangles from hair or blending colours or mixtures.

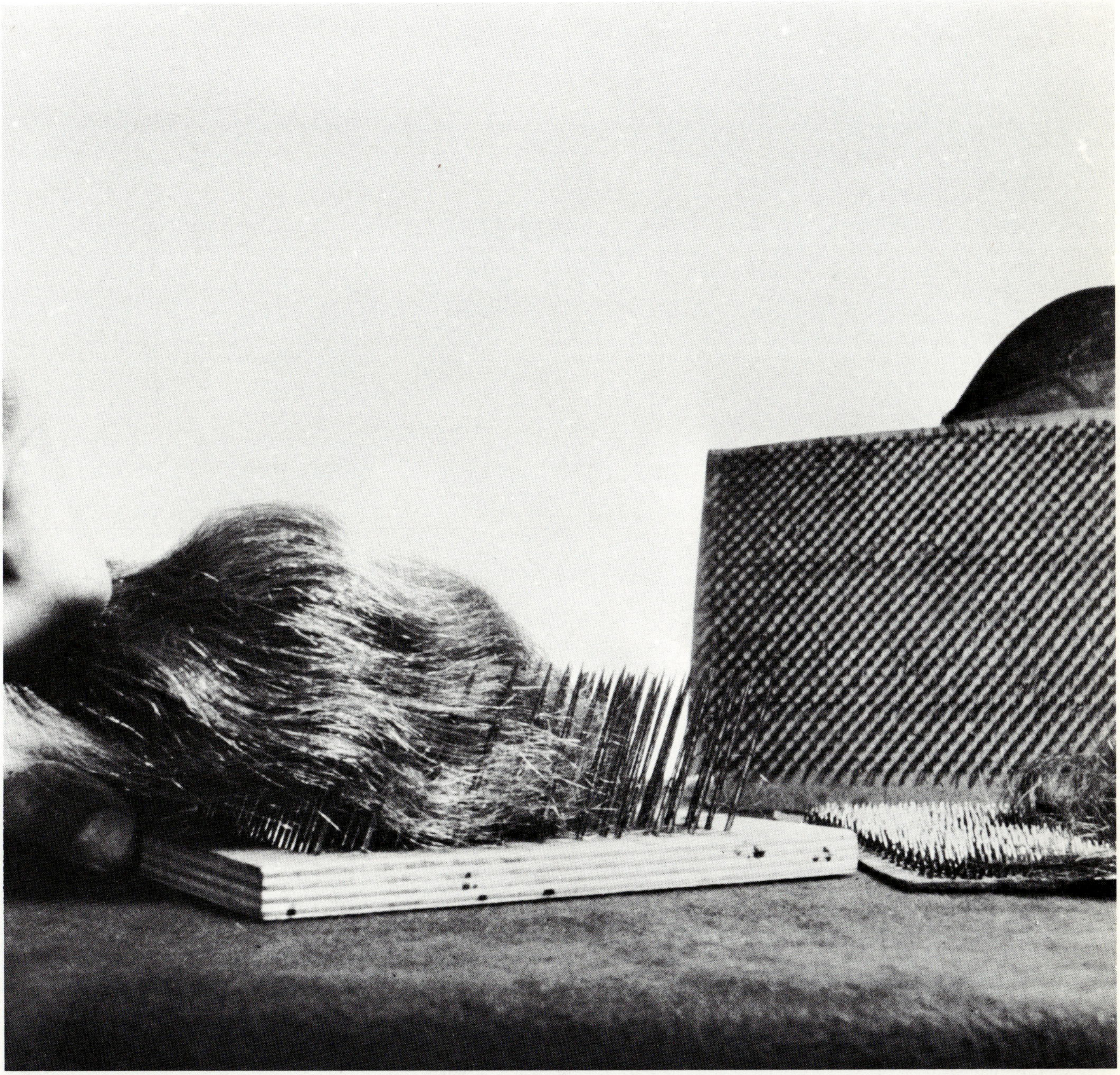

73 First and most important—all tangles are removed from the hair first with a brush, hackle or wide-toothed comb.

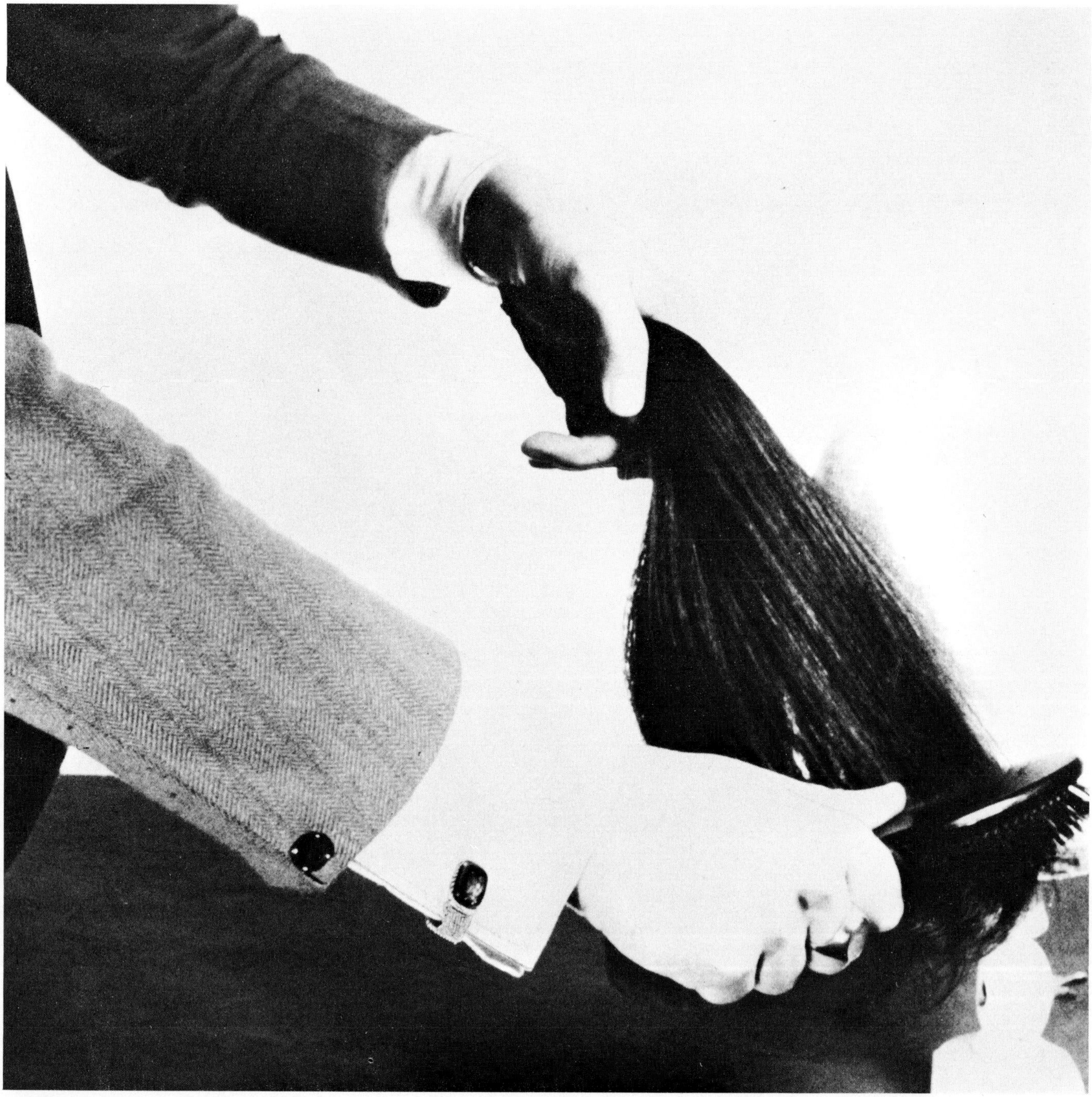

piece is then put into a large bowl. (If mixing a shampoo solution do not overdo the proportion of shampoo. Otherwise it will be difficult to remove completely and will leave a dull film on the hair.)

The hair is then dipped into the solution, working in the lather gently with the hand. Never rub or the hair will quickly tangle.

The piece is plunged gently up and down in the solution, working in the lather along the entire hair length. This is repeated until all the dirt and grease disappear. The solution must be renewed for an extra dirty piece.

The photographs on the next two pages illustrate these operations.

Next comes rinsing under a running tap in warm—not hot—water from the base downwards. The water is cupped in the palm and worked through the hair. This is continued until every trace of shampoo has been rinsed away.

The special solution has a built-in conditioner but an ordinary shampoo should be followed by a conditioner, to restore initial hair sheen and remove possible tangles.

Restoring condition

A liquid-type conditioner is put into a bowl and the hair immersed in it. Then the conditioner is gently combed into the hair, starting at the ends and working upwards to the roots. If the hair still tends to tangle, it should be re-dipped in the conditioner and combing continued until the hair runs free.

Rinsing is the same as for shampooing, from the base downwards. Surplus moisture is dispersed by pat-drying with a towel, never rubbing. The piece is then ready for drying. Some people advocate hanging up to dry naturally and then re-dampening for setting. Others advise setting right away and drying under a hot dryer for up to four hours. It all depends on the type of hair and you should check with your supplier first.

74 With the base held firmly in one hand, the hair is dipped in the solution and the lather worked gently in along the entire hair length with the other hand.

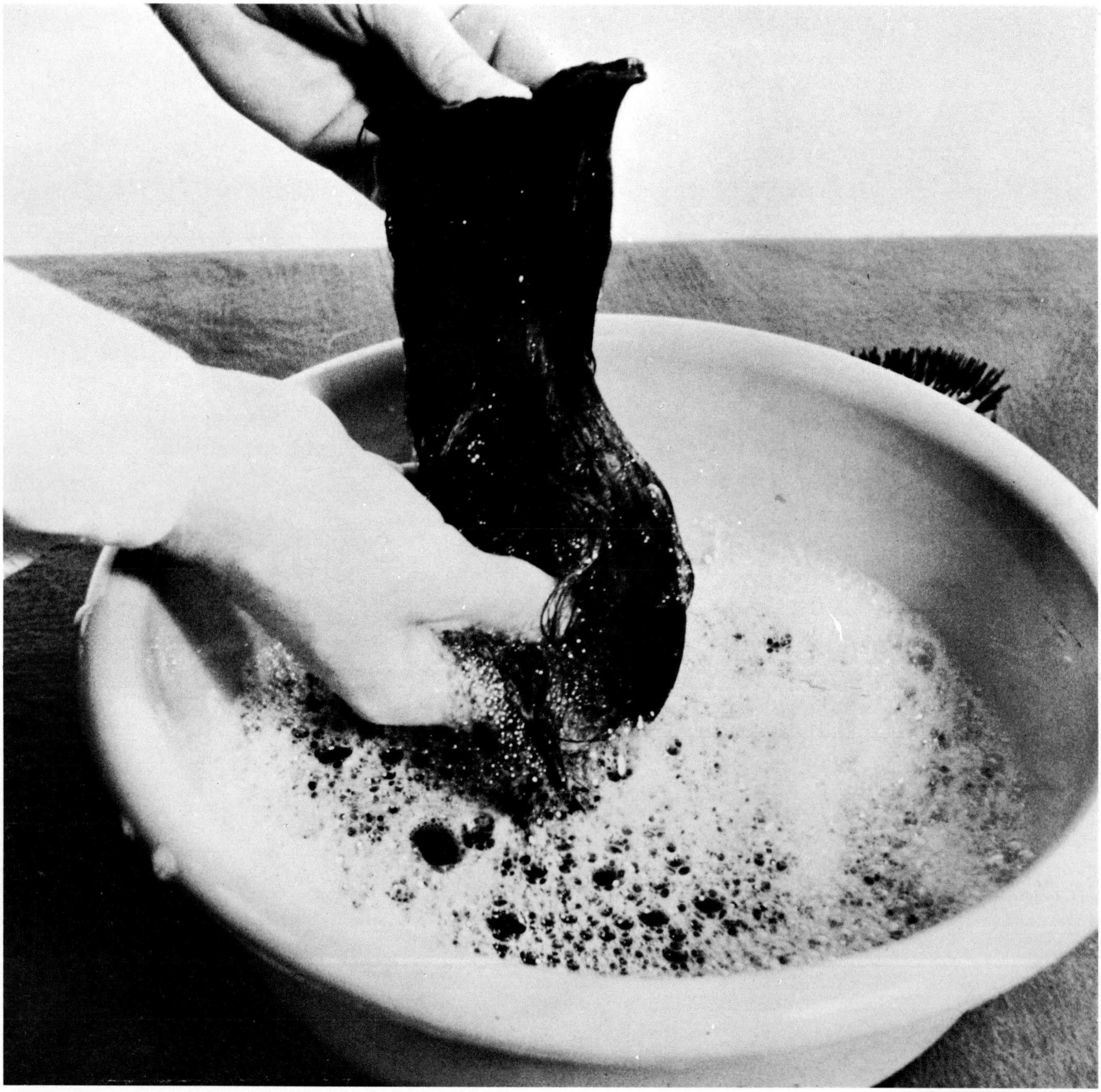

75 Gentle plunging in and out of the solution is continued until all dirt and grease have disappeared.

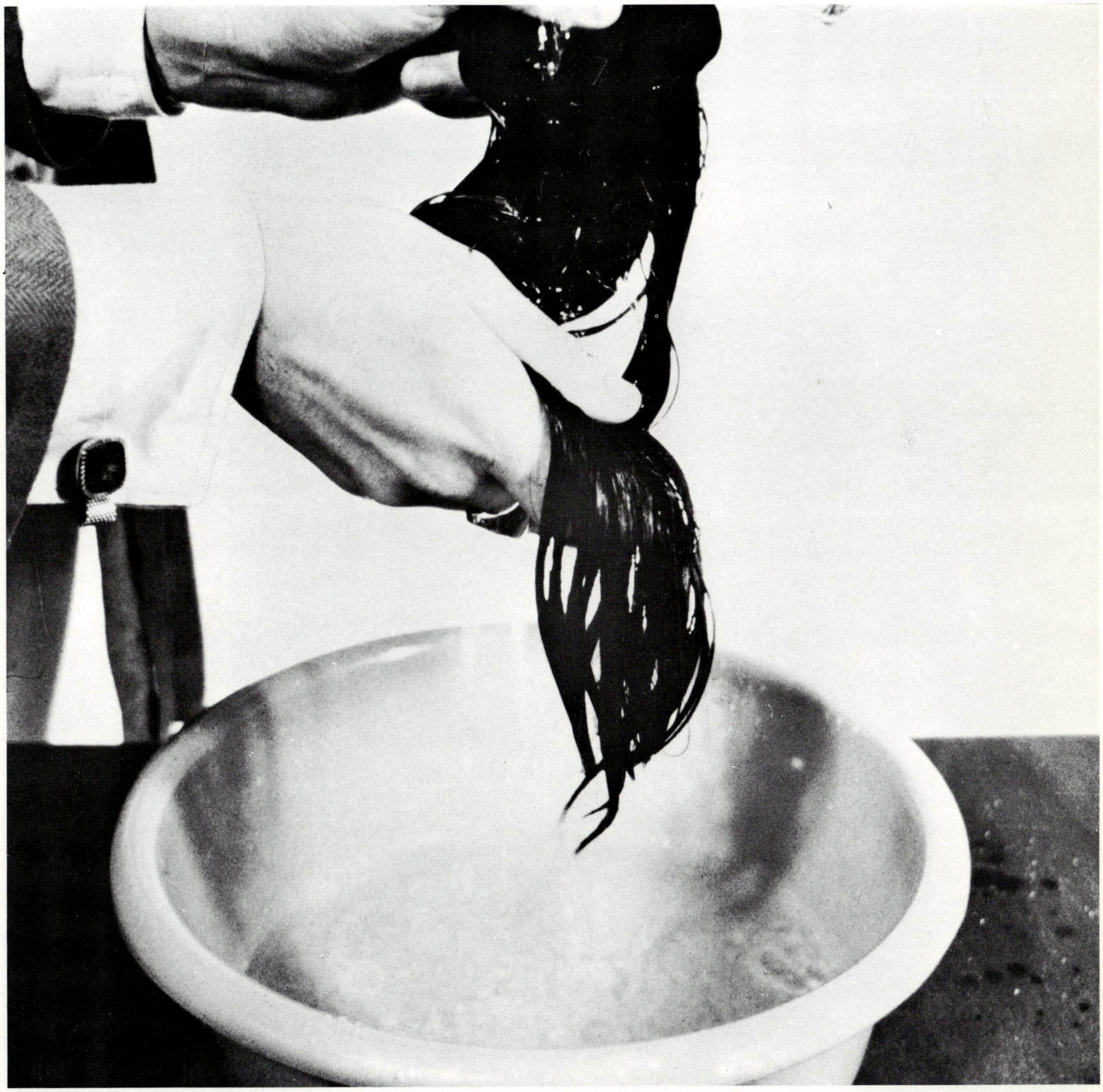

Professional Servicing—Colouring Hair

The permanent type

The Brush-on Way

Permanent hair colouring can be used successfully on Asian and European wigs and hairpieces, but only with skilled application and on quality pieces. Both the hair *and* the base must be first-class before a decision to colour is made. Inferior pieces often consist of a blend of hair and fibre. Avoid colouring these at all costs or you will end up with marked colour variations. Even if you are reasonably satisfied with the standards of the piece, appearances can be misleading. So be cautious and always colour test a hair cutting or mesh first.

Drastic colour changes should never be attempted. Only up to a difference of three shades is safe. Extra careful application is also essential. Colour must *never* be allowed to saturate the foundation or it will tend to rot it. Also, above all, the strength of the hydrogen peroxide additive must be kept as low as possible. Fake hair is more porous than the natural variety, therefore timing can be unpredictable. This, of course, means more frequent checking of development.

There are three ways to apply cream or liquid permanent colour—by brush, applicator, or with the dip method. Here, step-by-step, is the correct method of applying a cream-type product with a brush:

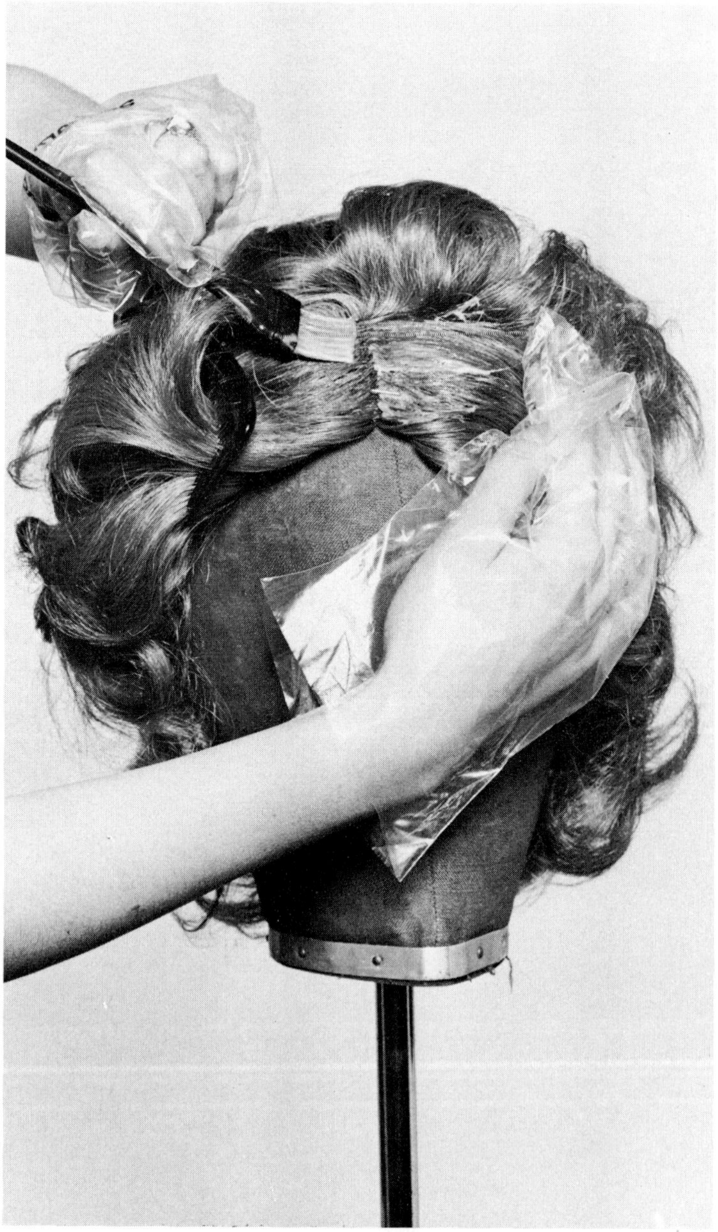

76 First—sectioning. The wig is divided into four and each dividing line marked with colour. One line will run from centre forehead to nape, the other from earpiece to earpiece. Starting point—the front hair is parted centrally and colour marking begun.

77 Using a comb to hold back the hair, sectioning with colour is then continued up and over the back of the wig . . .

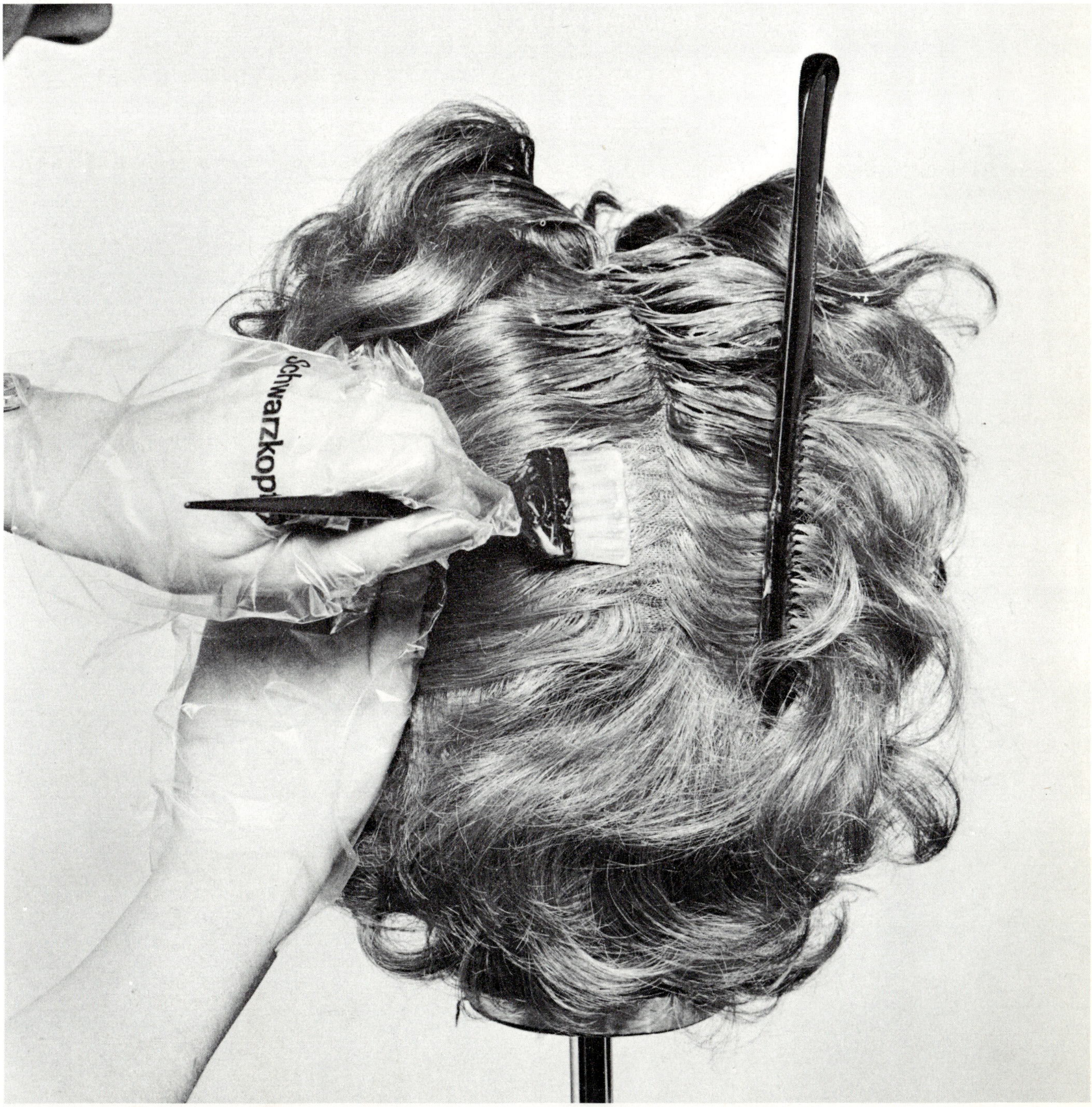

78 . . . until the line extends down to the hairline at centre nape.

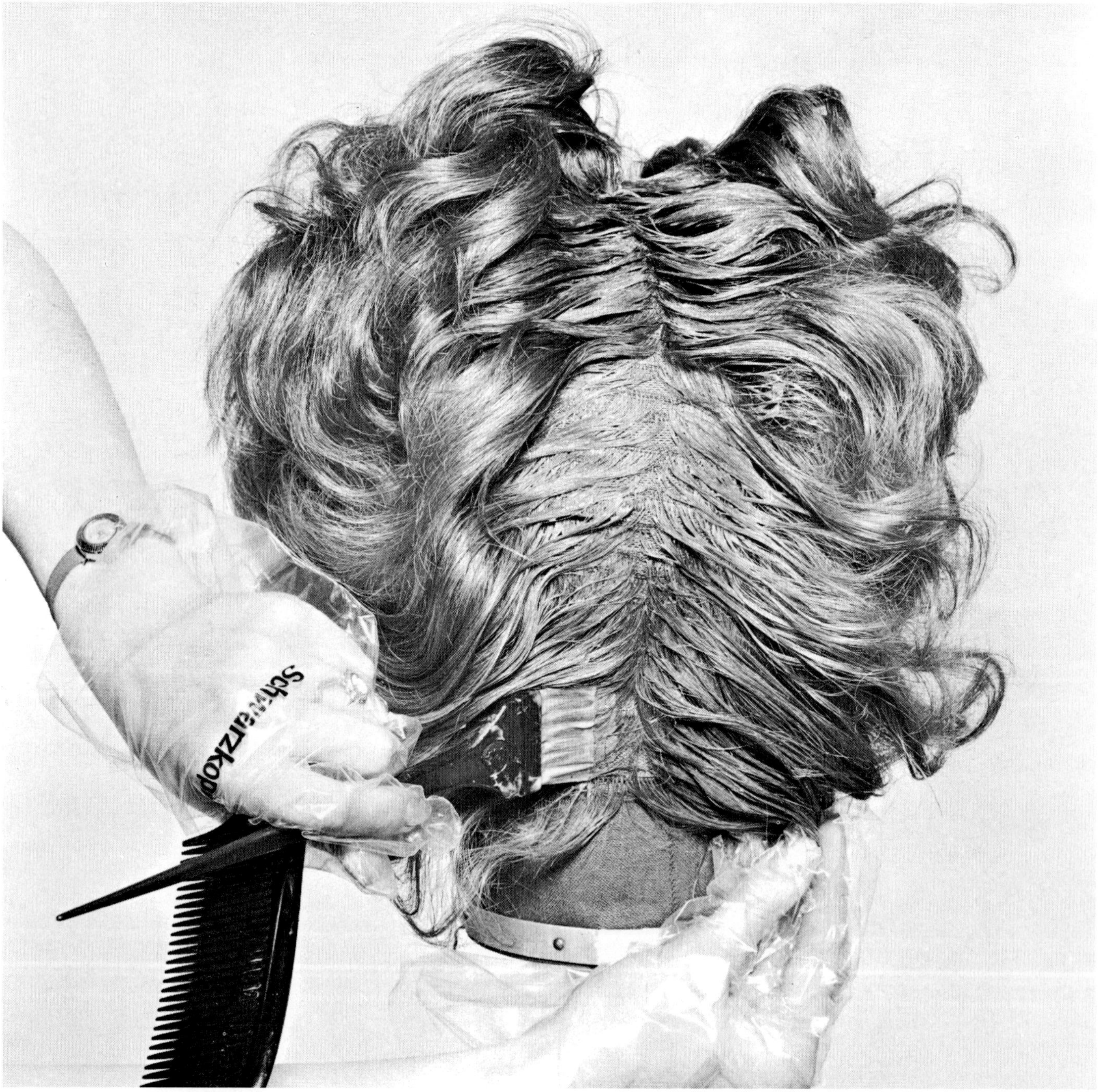

79 Now comes the side-to-side division. The hair is first parted at the crown and sectioned from either side just behind the earpieces. Again the line is marked with colour . . .

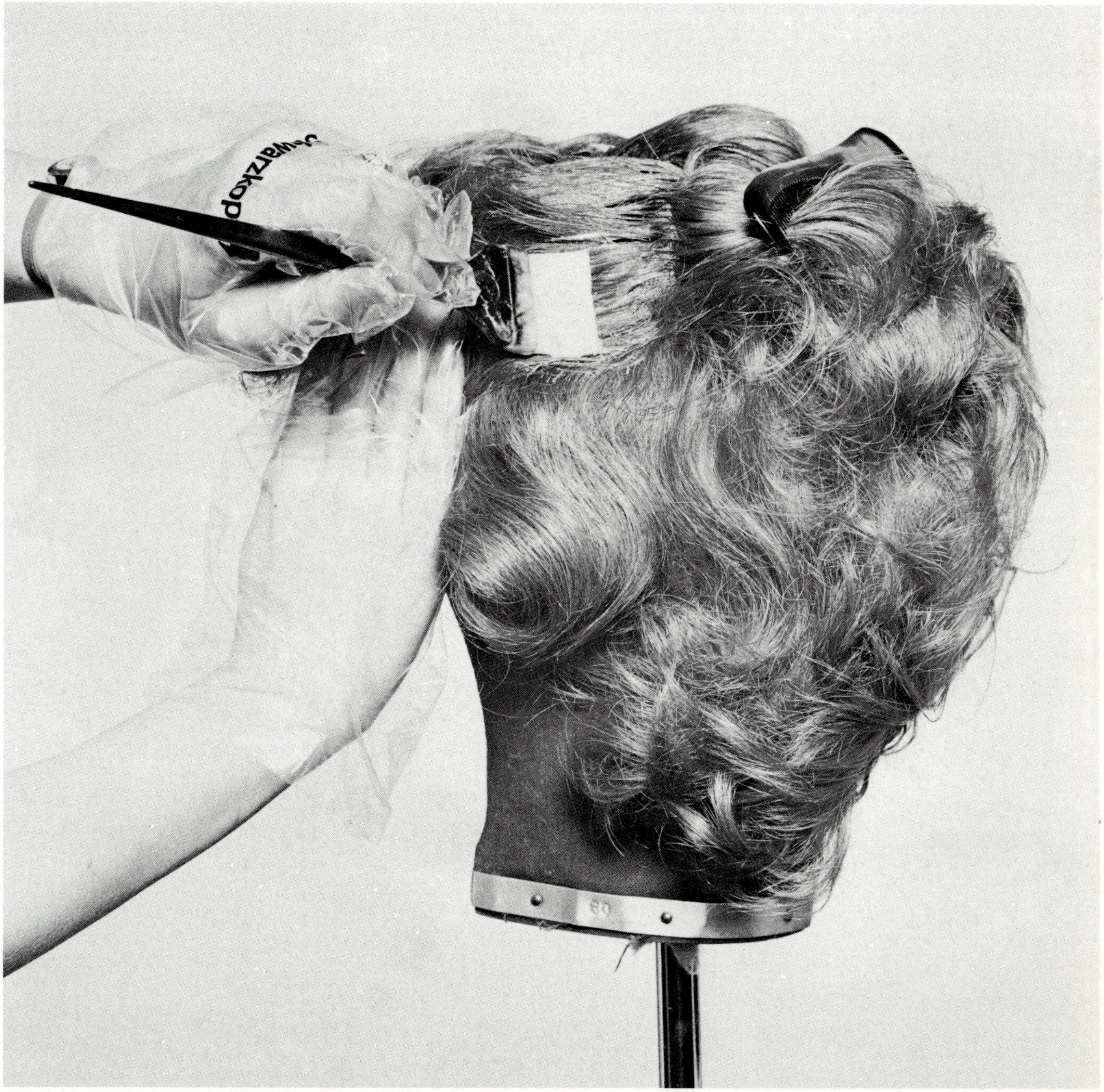

80 . . . and taken down to the hairline on either side of the head.

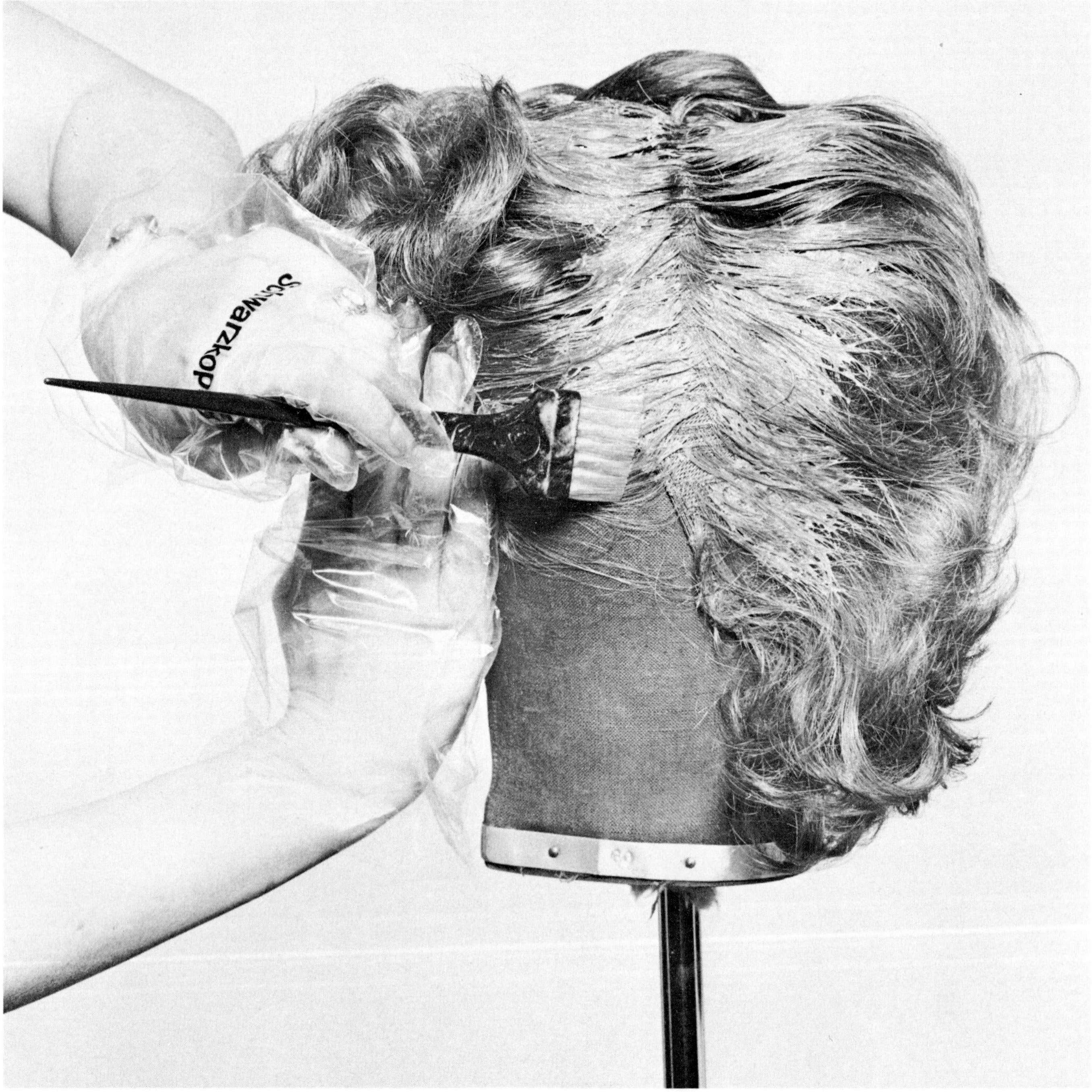

81 Next stage—filling in the sections. Colour is applied along the weft and brushed well into the hair from roots to ends.

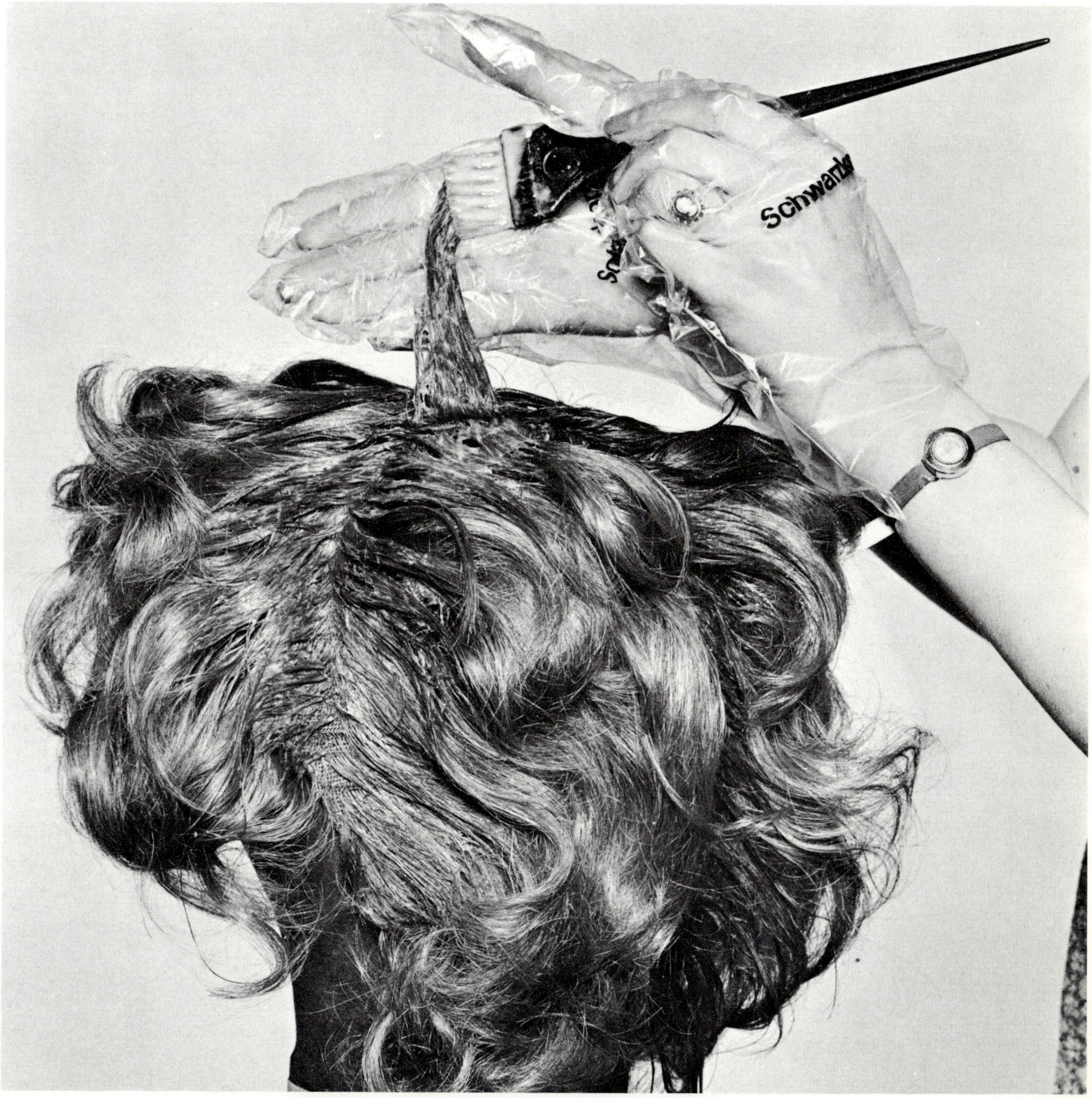

82 Colour is taken up to, but not on to, the foundation. And all colour overlap should be avoided.

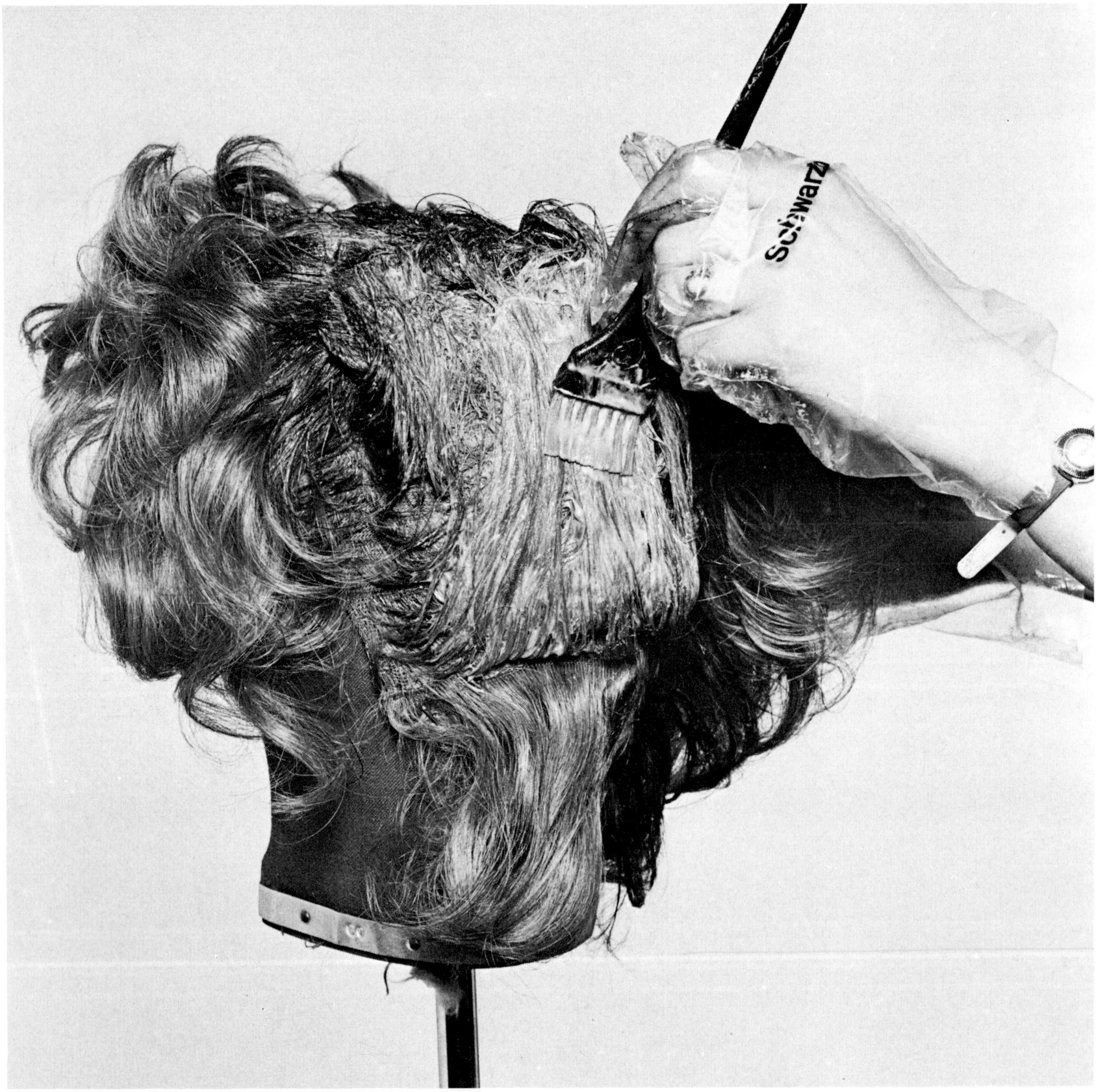

83 When all the hair has been coloured, a final check is made all round the hairline to see that no portion has been missed, particularly at the front as this part is the most noticeable.

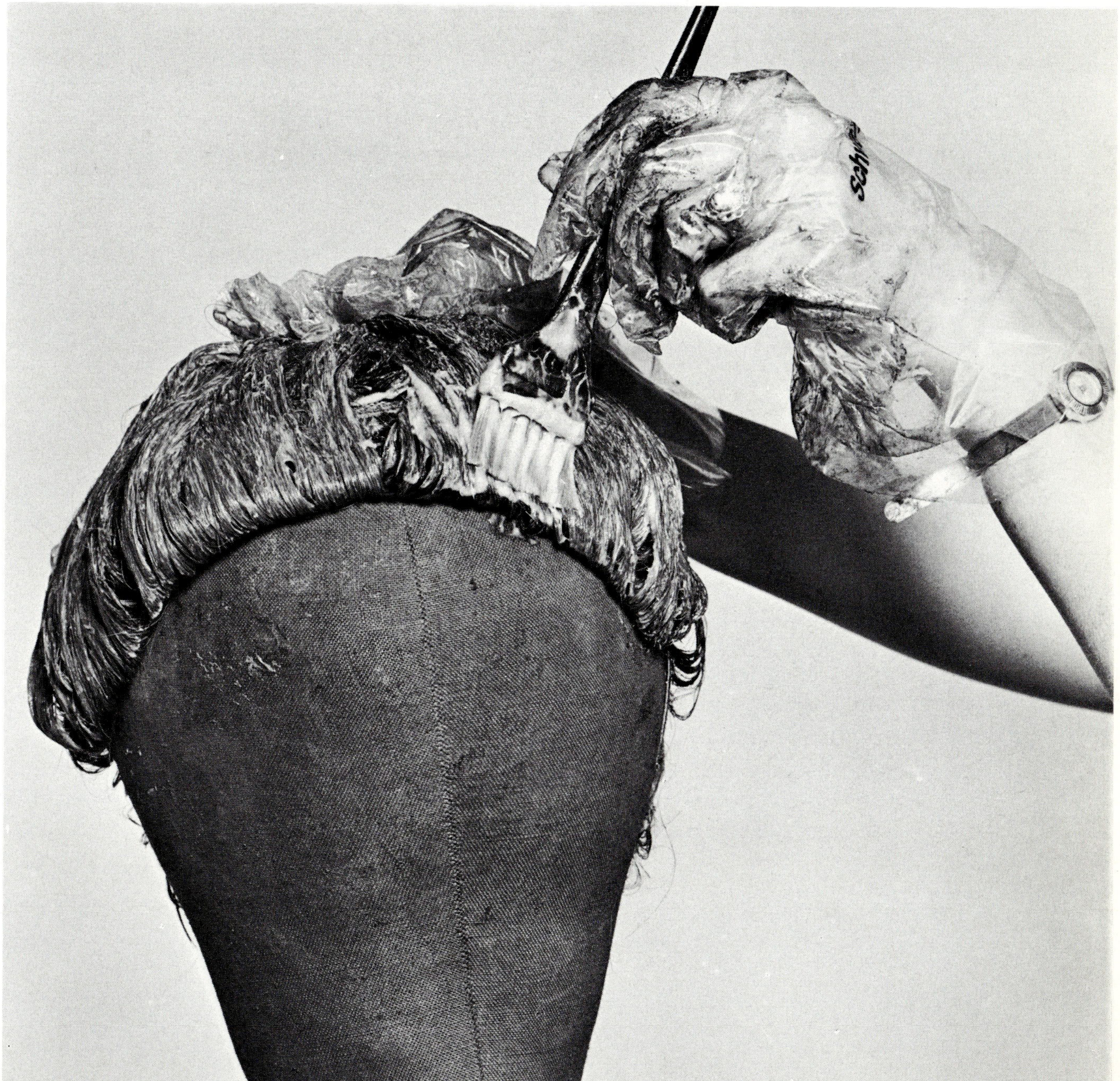

84 A final comb-through of colour to ensure complete penetration. It is then left to develop. Afterwards the wig, still pinned to the block, is rinsed under running water until it runs clear. After pat-drying with a towel, the wig is ready for setting and should be left on the block to dry out. It should never be removed from the block until completely dry to avoid possible shrinkage of the foundation.

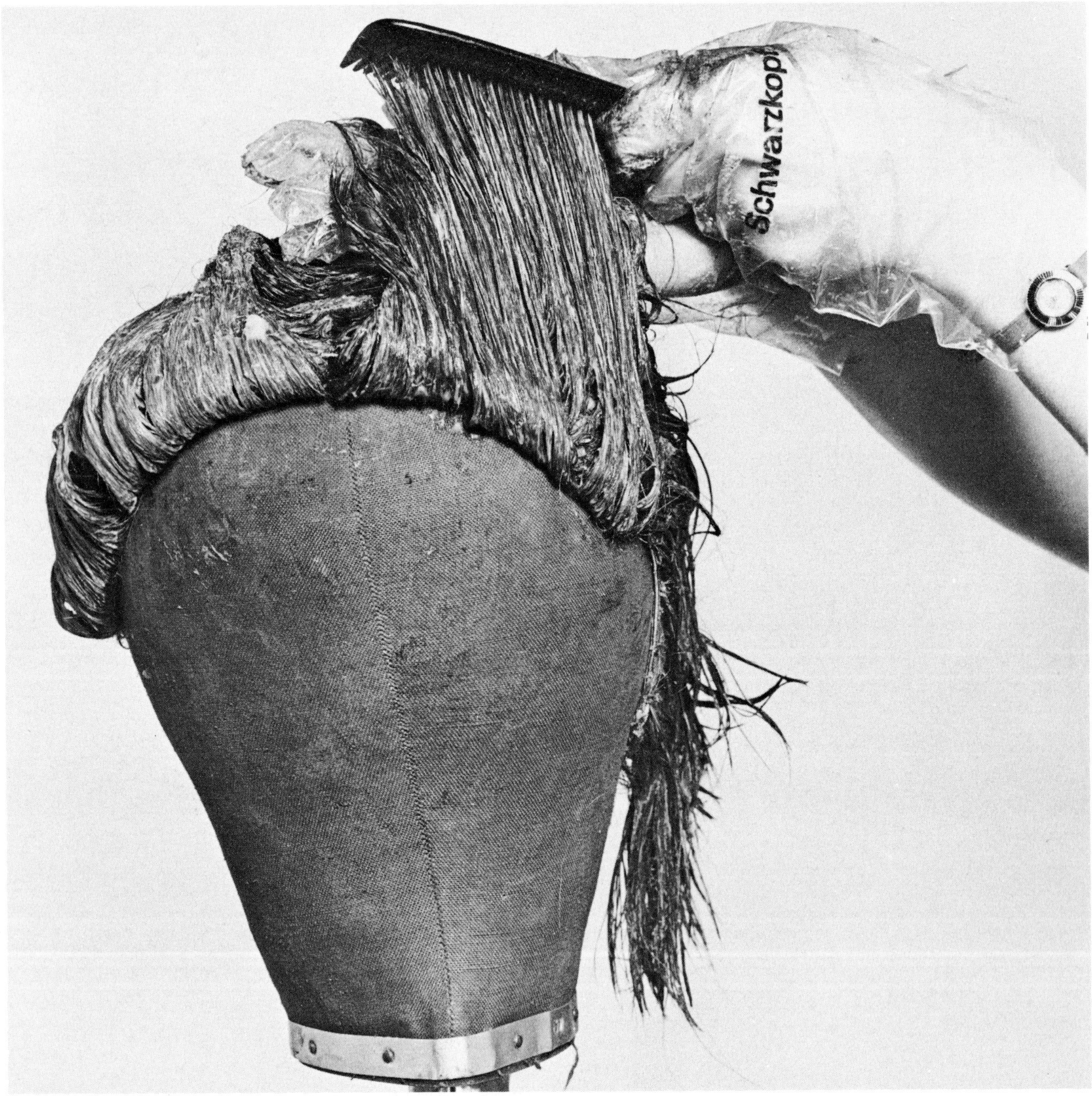

85 Transformation—a faded, lifeless wig now glowing with new colour and sheen.

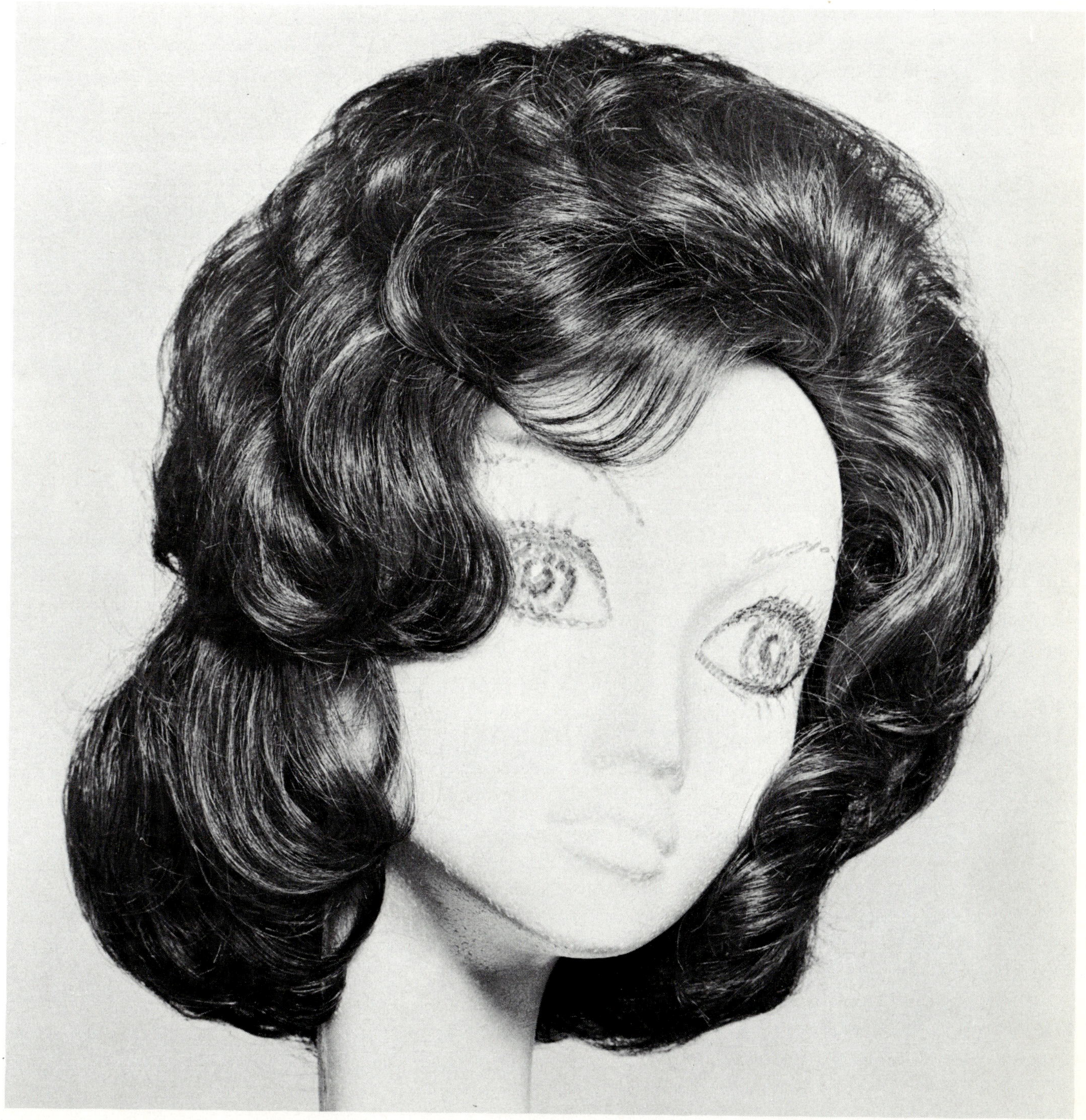

The Dip Method

The quickest and easiest way to apply long-lasting colour is by the dip method, using a permanent colour produced specially for wigs and hairpieces. First mix the solution according to the maker's instructions. Then pour it into a *non-metallic* container large enough to take the full length of hair. Holding the base firmly in one hand, dip the piece into the solution. Keep plunging it up and down in the liquid, working the colour into the hair with one hand. Repeat until all the hair has been covered. Check the base to see that the colour has penetrated evenly. Otherwise it will come out patchy and look unprofessional.

Next immerse the whole of the piece again in the solution. Turn it over several times. Then leave it to develop. Check after ten minutes by rubbing the hair with a piece of cotton wool. Normally it will take about thirty minutes to process. If the hair is extra porous, though, it can take up to two hours. This is because, although porous hair absorbs colour quicker, it does not retain it and, therefore, requires a longer development time.

After processing is completed, lift the piece out of the solution. Press out the surplus colour and rinse thoroughly. For a hairpiece, hang it up to dry out naturally. For a wig, pin it on a correct size block and leave to dry.

The semi-permanent type

Semi-permanent hair colouring is child's play to apply to natural hair. However, when it comes to using it on Asian hair, then the problems start. First, the piece can consist of several types of hair woven together and each will react differently to colour. Second, all raw Asian hair is heavily pre-processed and re-dyed with textile dyes. So any hair shade can result. Third, the extent of the various pre-processing can vary from piece to piece, as well as within one design. This, then, is the formidable combination of unknown factors to be borne in mind, especially for hairpieces expected to be an exact match for the owner's natural hair. Hairpieces or half-wigs, incidentally, should always be matched to the customer's *front* hair which is lighter than at the back.

To summarize, whatever the colouring method, all hair should be freshly cleaned first if it is especially dirty or greasy. Make sure that it is completely dry before starting. All tangles must also be removed, using a small hand hackle, wide-toothed comb or brush.

Always colour test, before you start, on a wider section of hair than for natural hair. This will ensure that any variation in hair mixtures is covered. Never use a metal bowl or container to hold a colourant. It can set up a reaction which could even change the shade. With semi-permanent colour, some hair might end up quite a bit lighter than the rest. In this case, pick out the lighter hairs and re-colour. You may even have to choose a different shade to blend in.

To find out whether a wig or hairpiece is extra porous, first wet the hair. Then run your finger along it. Exceptionally porous hair will feel slimy. A rougher feel means that the degree of porosity is lower.

Shades of grey or pepper-and-salt mixtures have a strong tendency to yellowing. Counteract this with a setting lotion, colour rinse or semi-permanent colour in a silver shade. Avoid metallic or ash overtones by choosing shades with more red in them than you would for natural hair.

Professional Servicing—Perming Hair

The cold wave method on Asian hair . . .

Wig styles, linked as they are to fashion trends, are always changing. It may be that a woman with a straight wig wants it re-styled into curls. Or after hard and constant wear, a wig may have become limp and lustreless and need revitalizing. In both these cases, perming can be the answer, either to produce lasting curls or waves or to merely restore former bounce and shine. Remember, however, never attempt a perm on anything but quality hair or you could end up with a tangled mass.

Because of the drastic pre-bleaching of Asian hair before it is made up into wigs, choose a gentle cold wave process specially formulated for *bleached* hair. Always test first, and don't forget to mark the test curl to avoid double processing later on. Use a plastic, stainless steel or anodized aluminium pin. Also bear in mind that Asian hair is considerably stronger and more porous than natural Western hair. This means quicker processing, so check after five or six minutes.

Sectioning, of course, varies from style to style but, wherever possible, it should be along the weft. Use medium-large curlers for winding the hair as a general rule; or large if processing is extra fast during testing. Winding should be firmer than for natural hair but take care to avoid pulling the hair too strongly and tearing the foundation.

. . . and untreated European hair

This stage-by-stage perming demonstration shows how to restore body and bounce to a much-worn hair wig. As the hair is untreated European, a gentle cosmetic conditioning body wave is used to produce natural looking movement of the hair. Sectioning is pre-planned to style. The extra-penetrating lotion means that the hair can be damped with water beforehand, making it easier to handle. It also speeds up winding as gloves need not be worn. Strong fibre end papers are advocated, as they hold the springy hair more firmly, and large-size curlers are right with this type of process.

The perm lotion is applied *twice* after winding to ensure complete penetration. Care must be taken to keep it off the foundation or it will tend to rot it. Then the hair is left to process, checking development after five or six minutes. After processing is complete, the wig, still wound in curlers and attached to the block, is rinsed thoroughly in running water. When the water runs clear, the hair is dabbed dry with a towel.

Next comes neutralizing, applying two-thirds of the neutralizer to the wound hair. Then the hair is taken out of the curlers and soaked again with the remaining third of the neutralizer. With most perms the neutralizer has to be rinsed out of the hair but with this type it does not. The hair can then be set.

Illustrations 86 to 94 on the following pages show these operations in detail.

86 The aim was to restore the original look—a casual, non-defined style with body and shining soft movement.

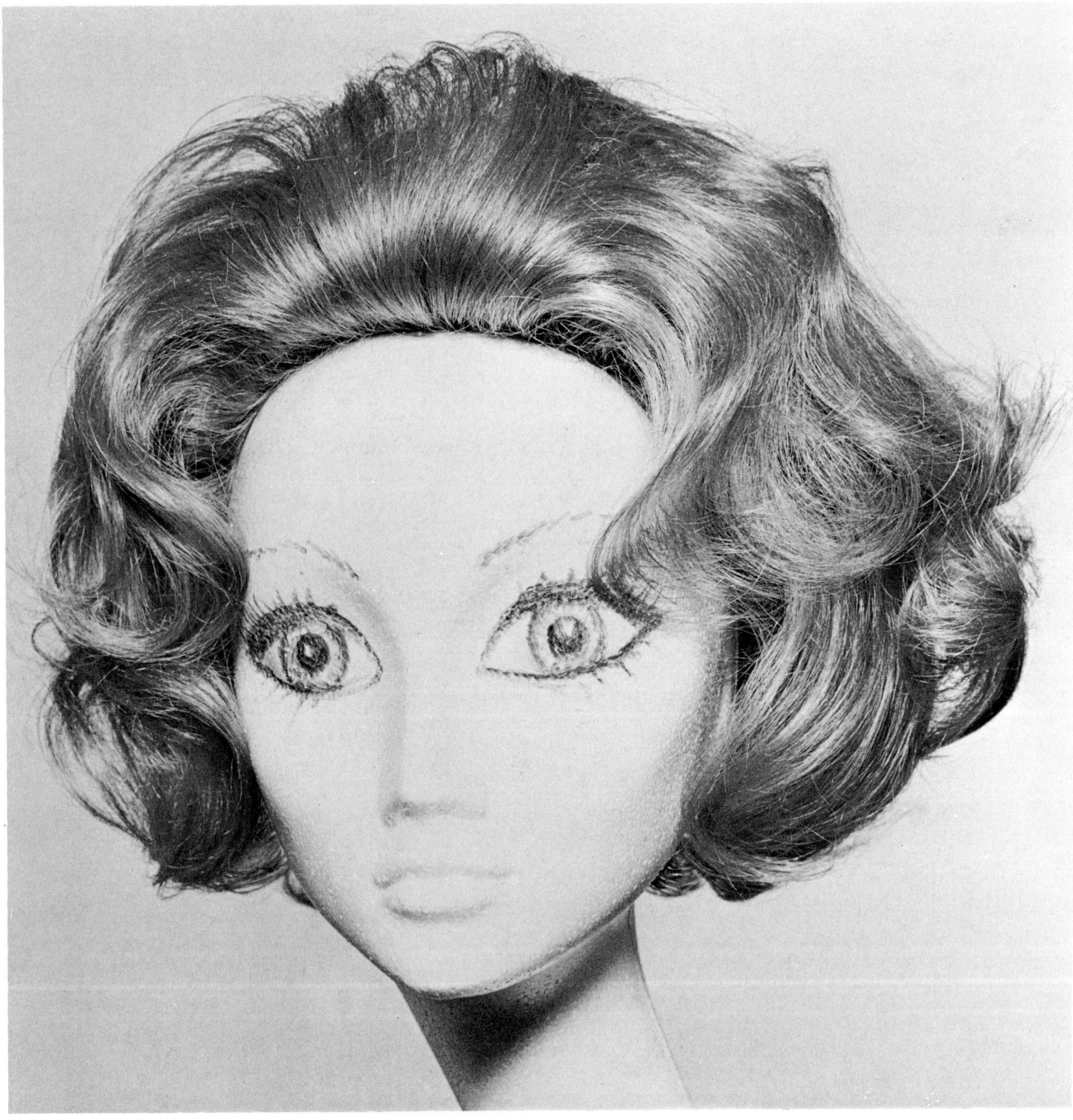

87 The sectioning pattern with the head divided into six—front and back sections plus two on each side.

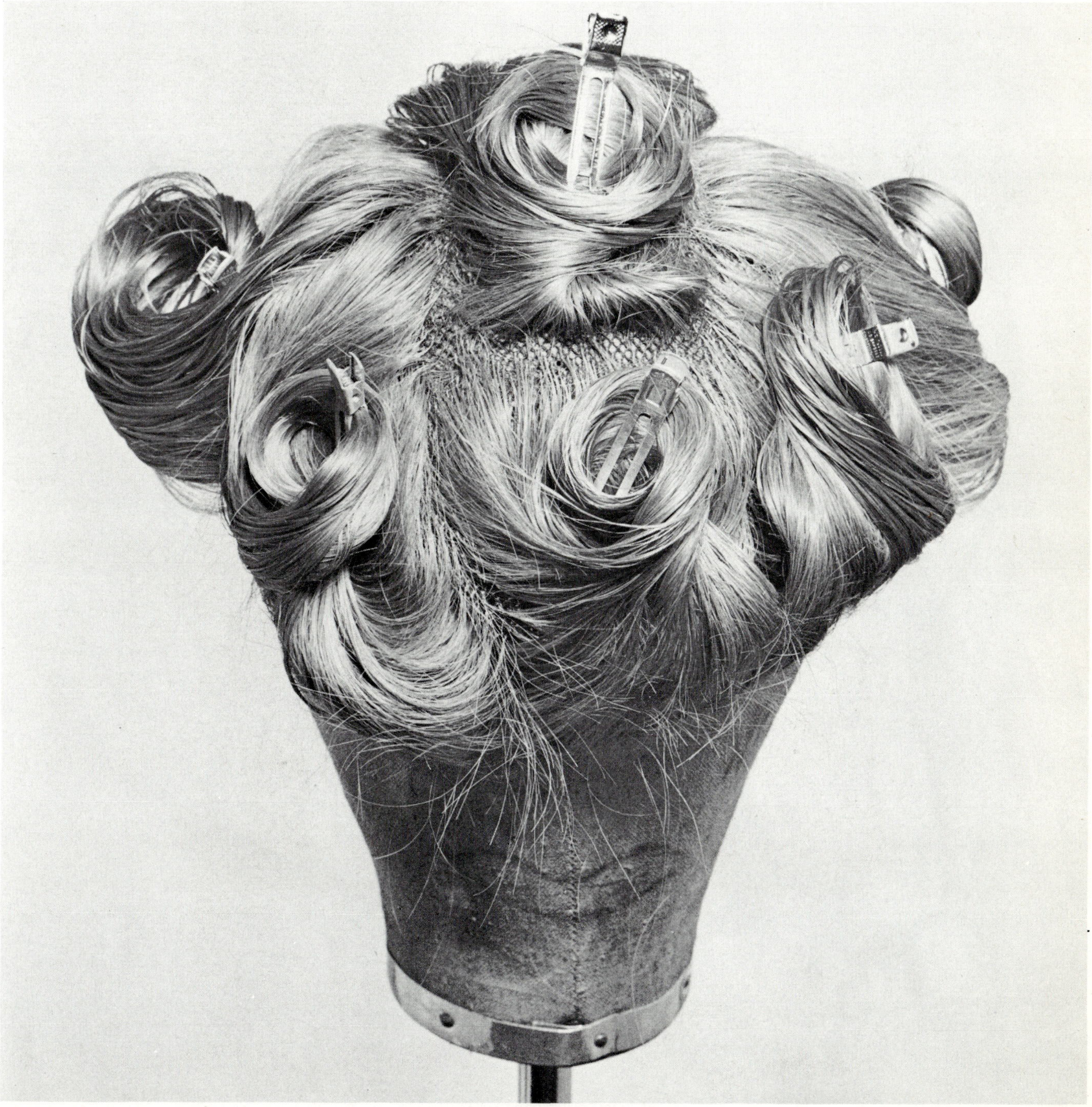

88 The amount of hair to be wound (the mesh) must always be the same width as the curlers, *never* larger.

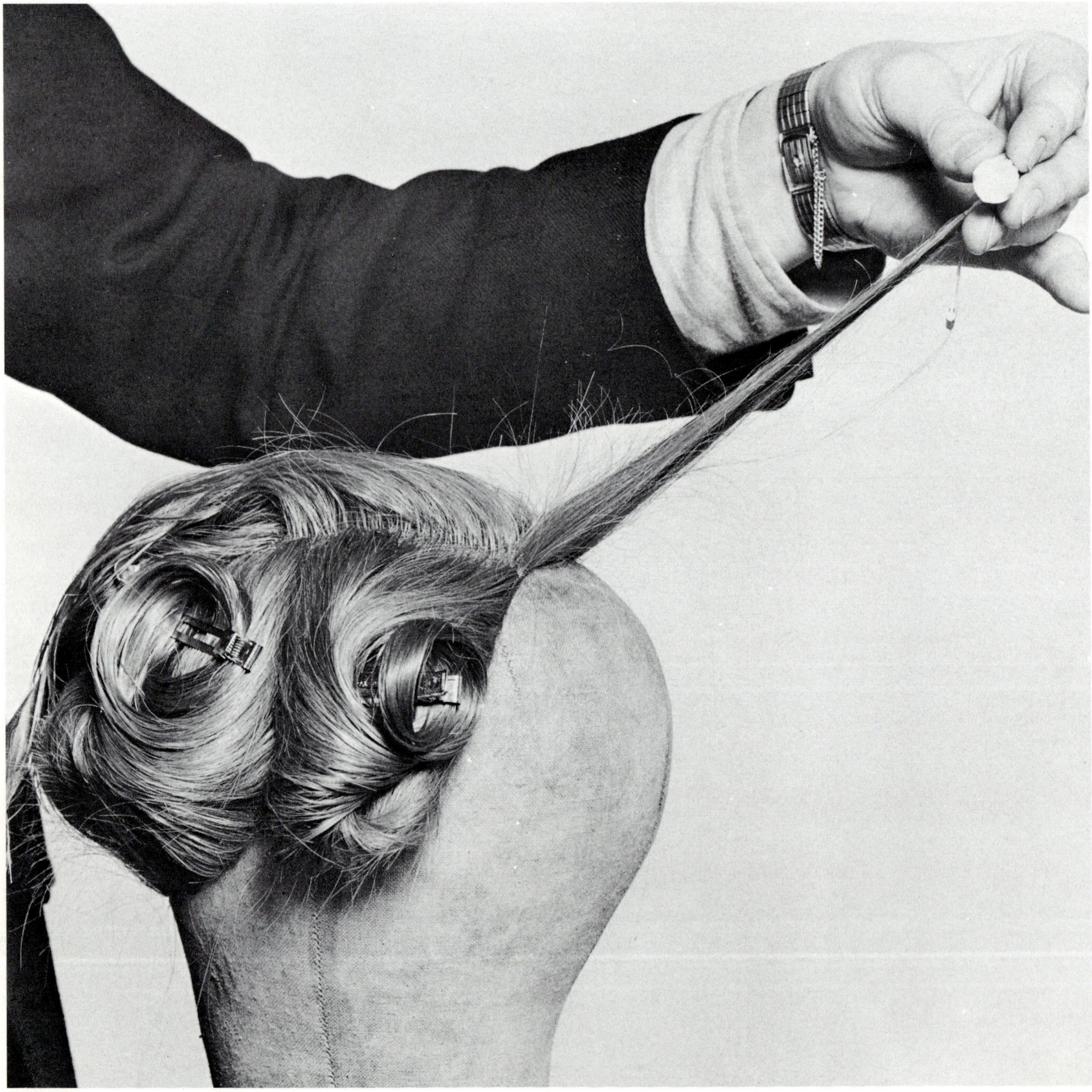

89 Precision winding on the top section—not easy with the springy hair. Curlers are wound firmly, but with tension spread evenly, avoiding hair breakage. Each curler sits on its own mesh ensuring that the wave is taken down to the hair roots.

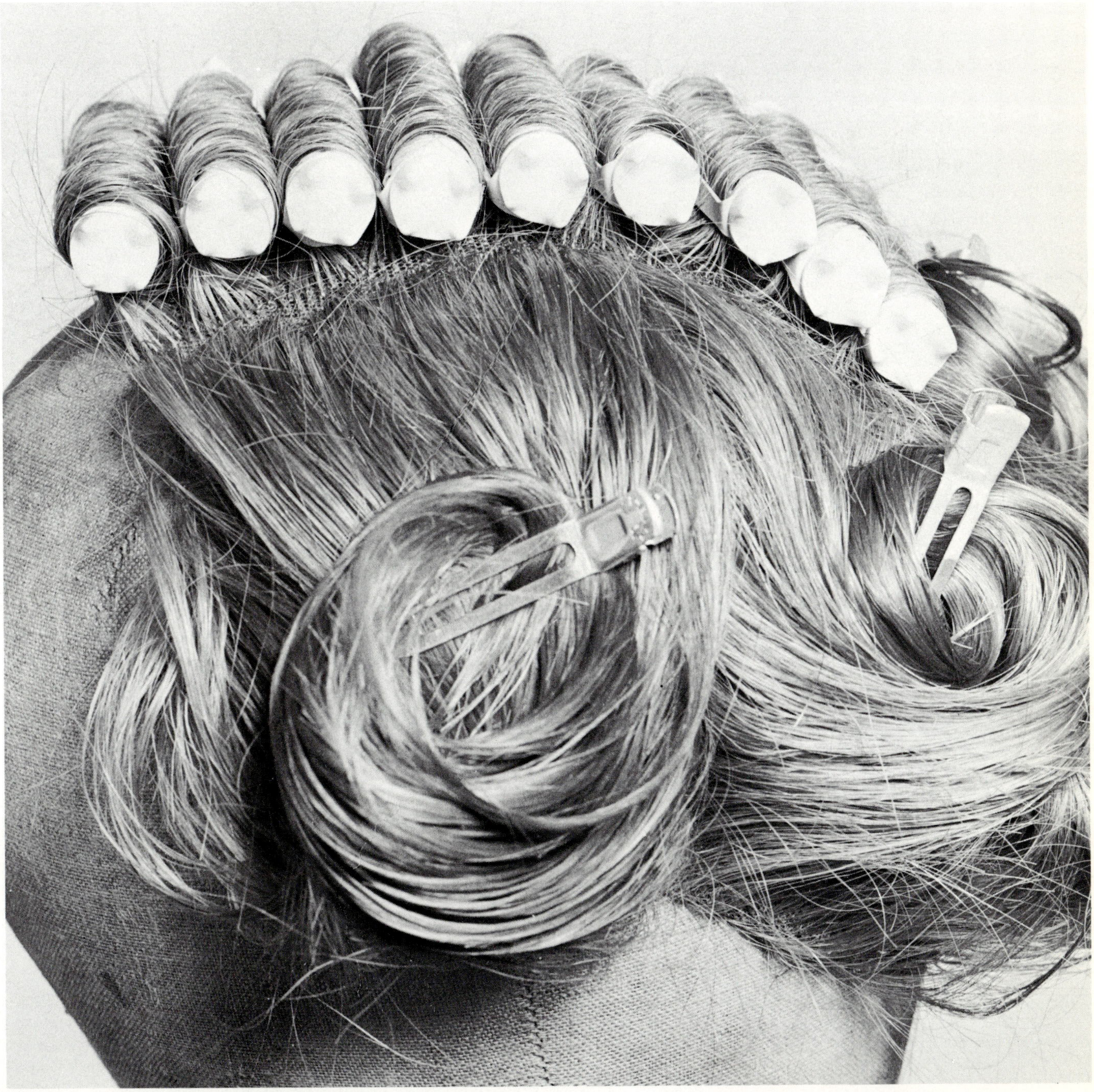

90 More meticulous winding continuing down the back section to the nape of the neck.

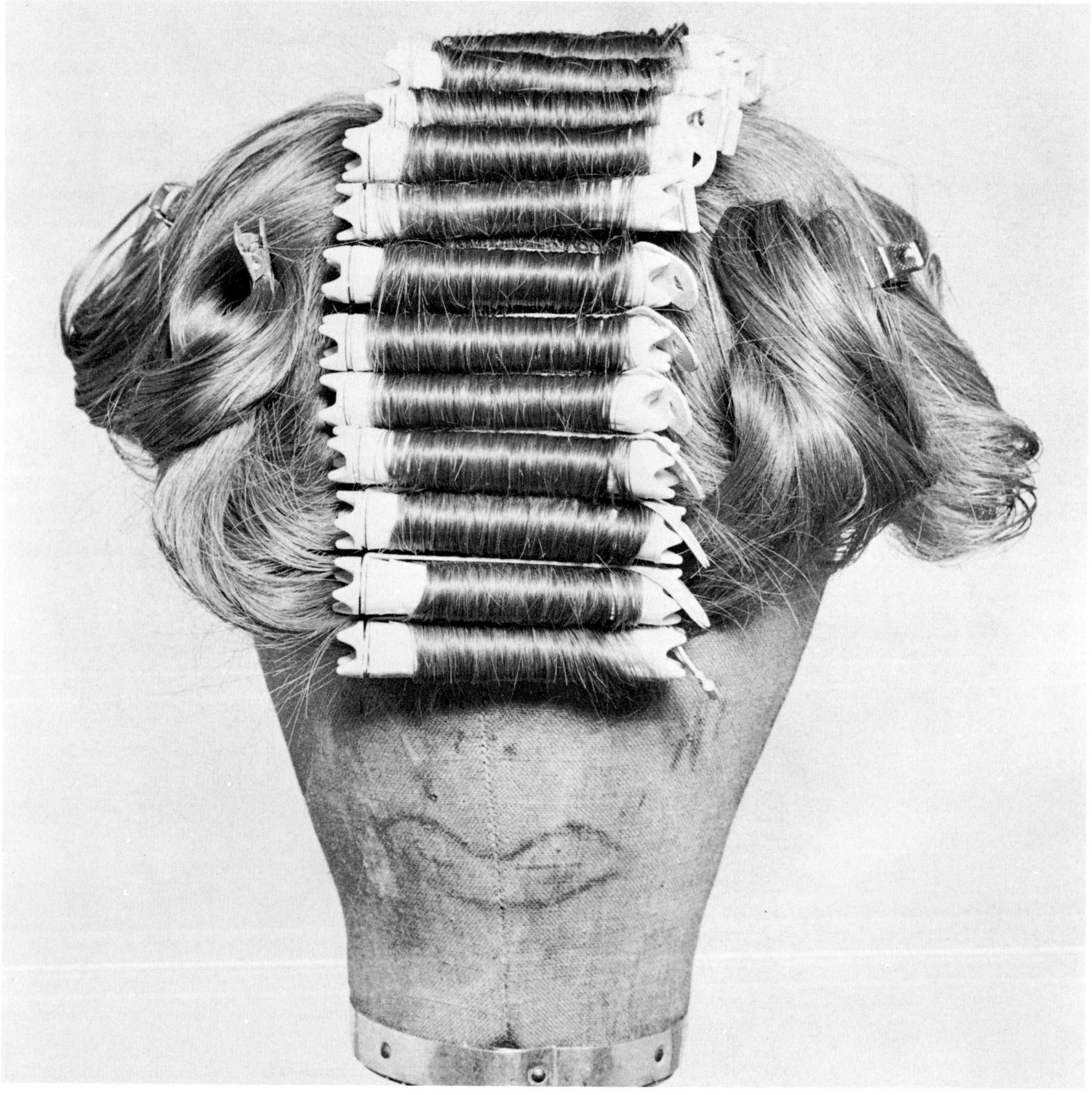

91 Next to be wound are the side back sections . . .

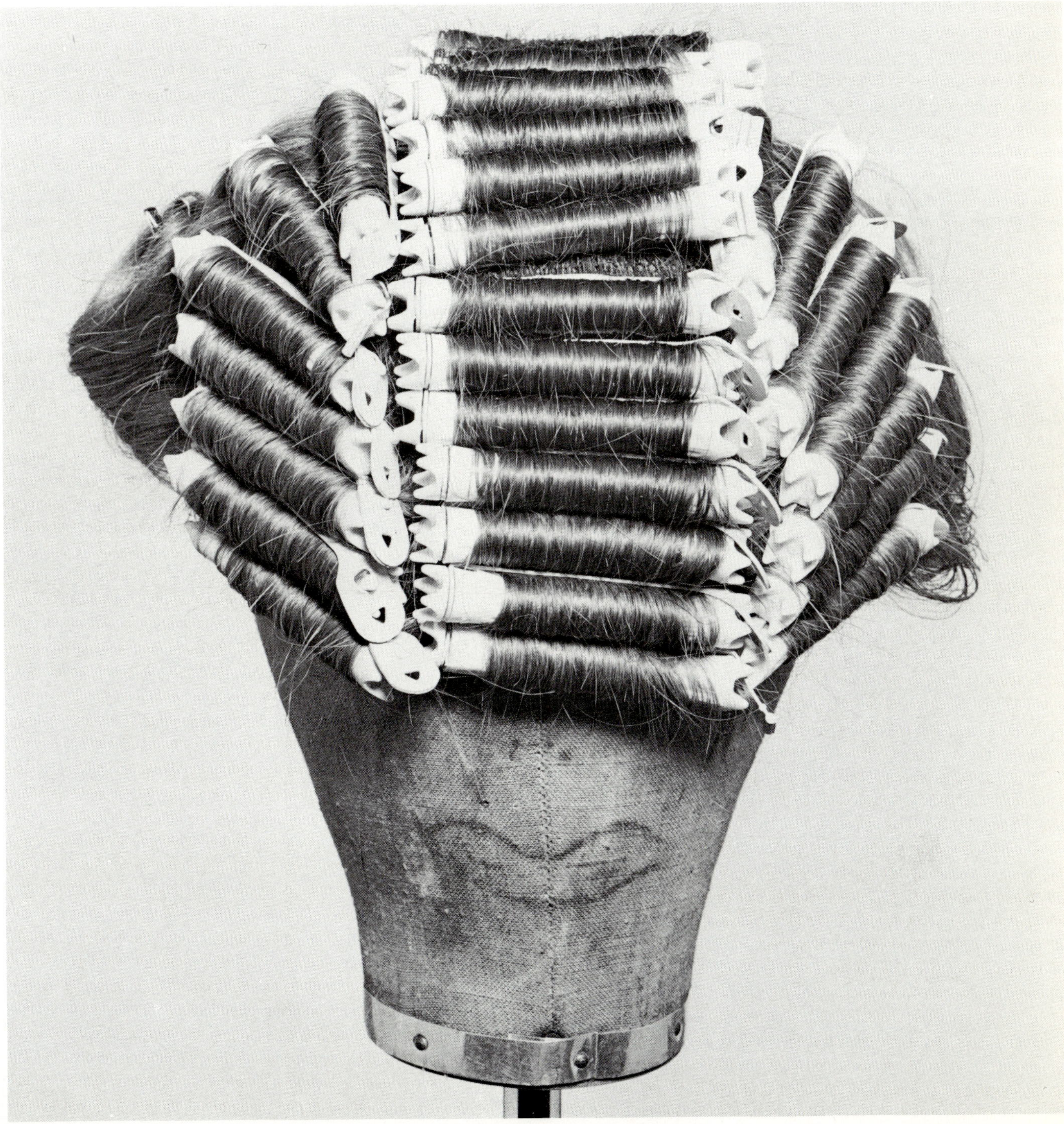

92 . . . and, finally, each of the front sides. Re-position the plastic pin marking the test curler if it becomes hidden during winding.

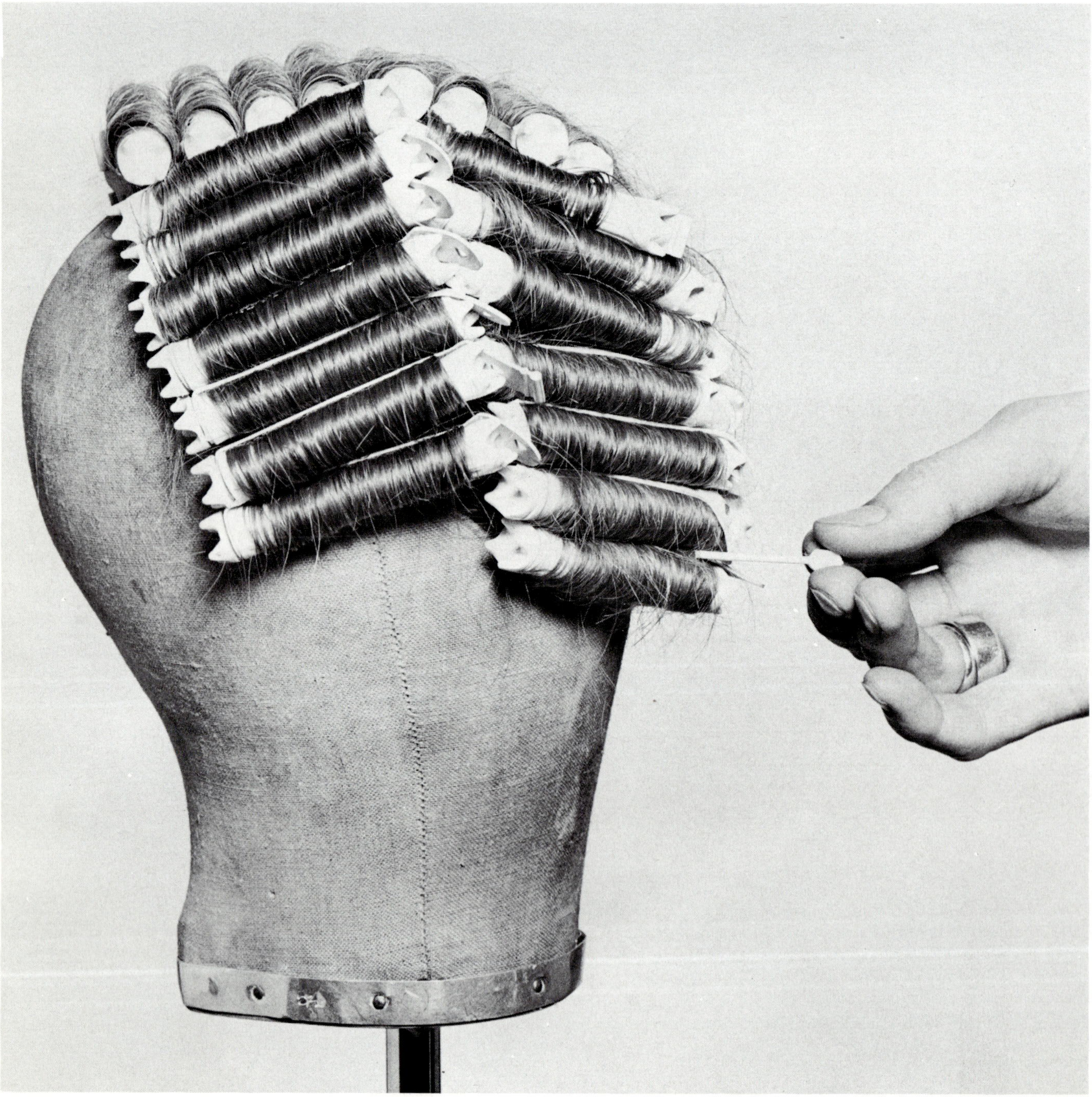

93 Next, applying the lotion to each curler. To prevent drips on the foundation, the forefinger is placed beneath each curler and used as a guide.

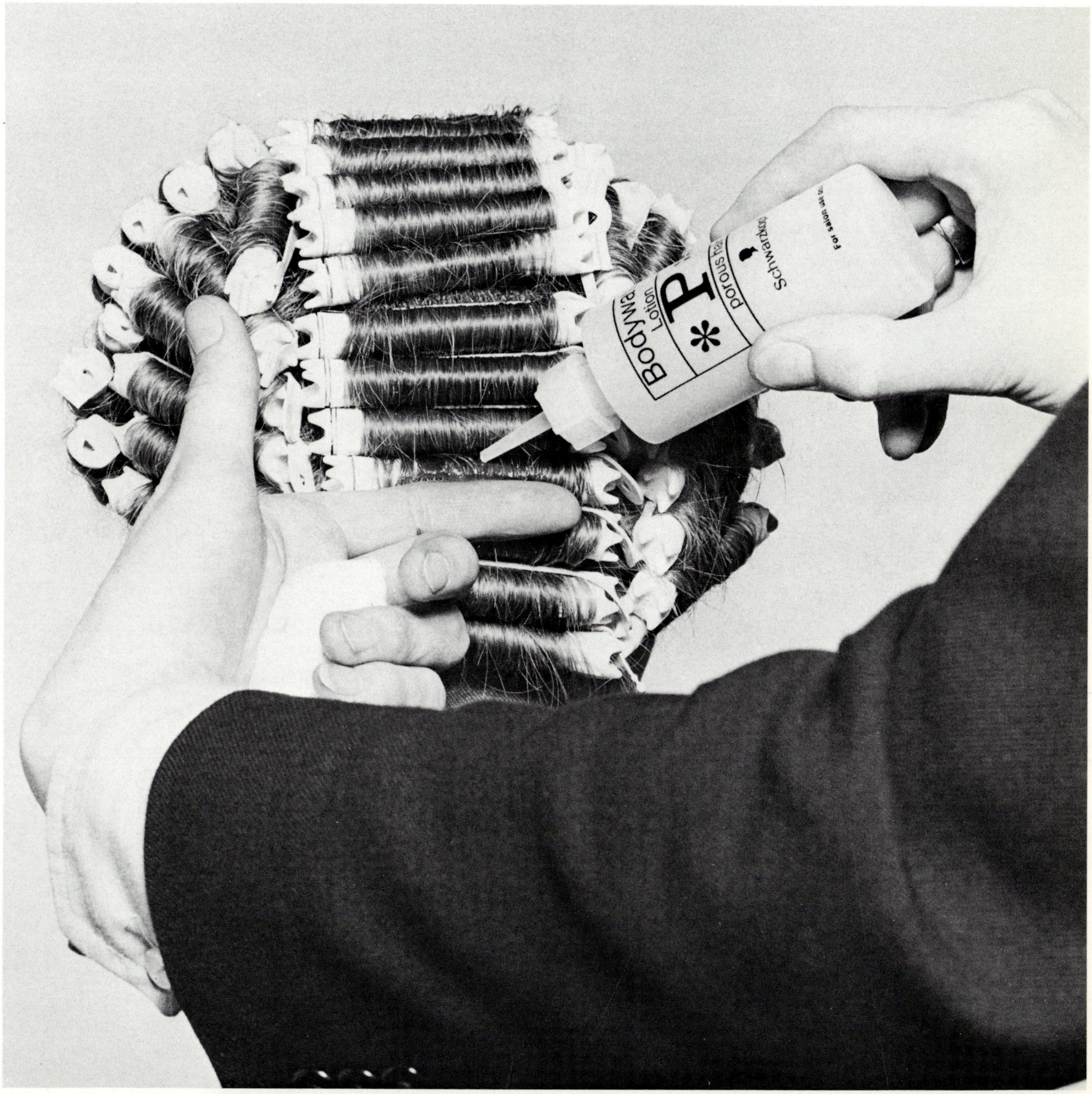

94 The correct degree of curl to aim for—with the wave going right down to the hair roots. The hair is then ready for setting after neutralizing and in this case does not need a setting lotion.

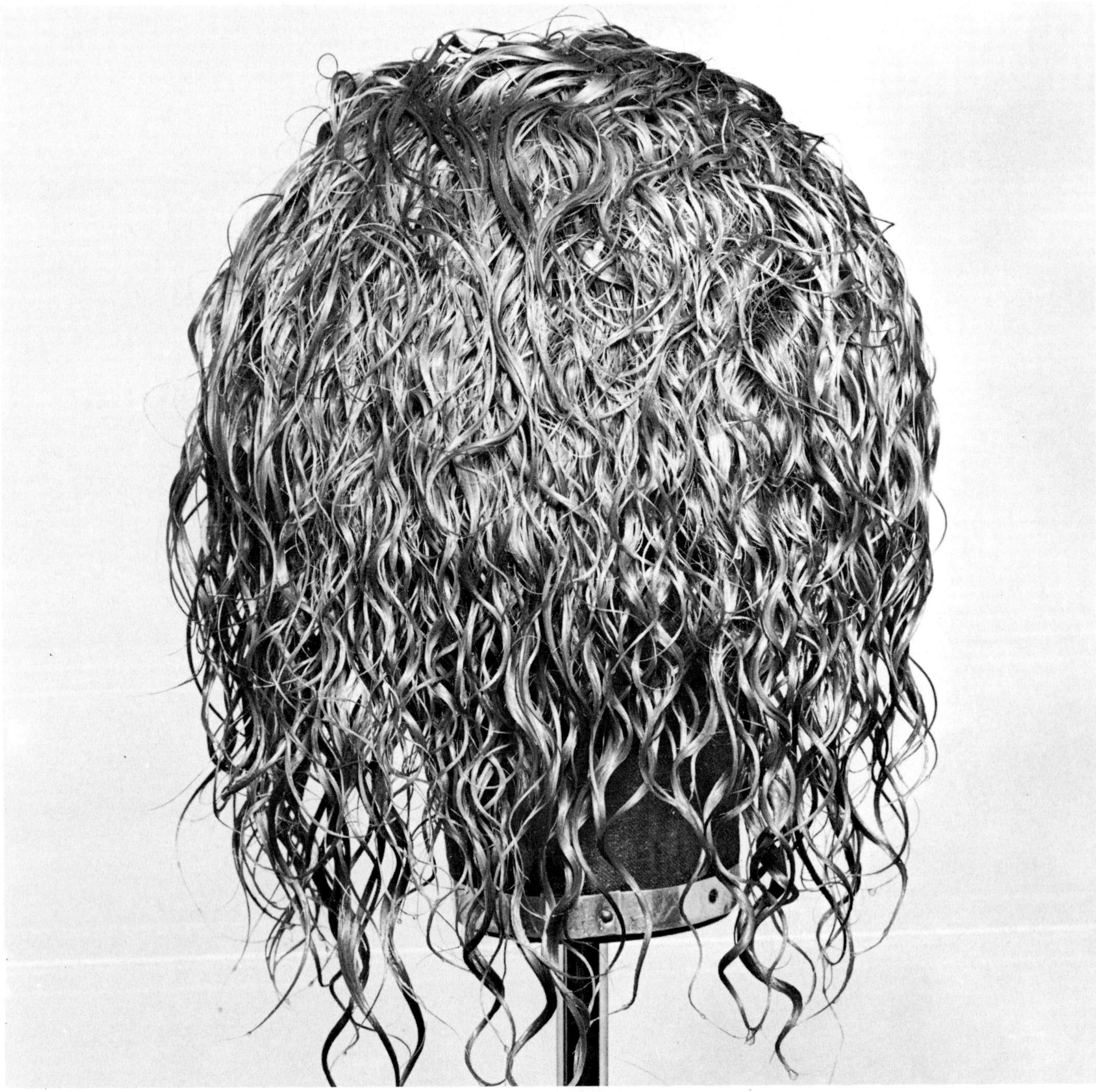

Perming by machine

Firm and lasting curls or waves can be achieved on Asian hair with a perming machine but, again, only on quality hair. The perm lotion should be oil-based, preferably with a built-in conditioner to make the hair more pliable and give it a sheen. Lotion strength should be based on the hair colour. The lighter the shade the weaker the solution, should be the rule. Asian hair is considerably more porous than natural hair and soaks up a lot more lotion. So make sure you have more than the usual amount to hand and apply it with a brush to ensure complete penetration.

Two applications are necessary—one before winding and the other after. If either is skimped, there is a danger of uneven processing. Again, the lotion must be kept off the foundation, or it will tend to rot it. When winding, take 3 cm (1 in.) sections of hair, no larger. Asian hair swells more than natural hair and, with a clamp-type machine, wider sectioning will not fit into the clamps. Use large-size curlers, otherwise the hair will frizz. Follow normal neutralizing procedure.

Acknowledgments

While this book was at the planning stage, I was greatly encouraged by the enthusiasm and help offered to me by leading firms within, and outside, the wig field. Their co-operation made the technical content of this book possible and I would like to record my deep appreciation to:

The Unilever Research Laboratories of Isleworth, Middlesex, for technical information and permission to reproduce their electron microscope photographs (Figures 8–13) and for *Clynol Ltd.* for arranging it.

Hair Plan,
for information and photographs of their wig factories in Hong Kong (Figures 20–25). Also *Wig Marla* for additional information.

Delbanco Meyer Wigs,
for arranging for Dolores Potter, their fashion adviser, to demonstrate razor-cutting and cutting-to-the-face techniques (Figures 52–71) and for the expertise of Maggie Dennis, former fashion adviser. Also for the company's permission to reproduce illustrated techniques and drawings from their training booklet (Figures 36–51).

Trend Products of Brighton,
for permission to reproduce sequences from their Teach-in programme which includes Figures 72–75, plus Sally Robinson's excellent drawings (Figures 3 and 4).

Schwarzkopf International Hair Cosmetic House,
for technical information and for arranging for technical manager, Ian Beavis, to demonstrate perming on a wig lent by Model Wigs (Figures 86–94), and Janet Richmond, studio technical consultant, to demonstrate colouring (Figures 76–85).

Fair Lady Fashion Wigs,
for supplying and extending permission to use Figure 16. This outstanding picture, copyright by the Paris fashion photographer, Ole Bjork, is also reproduced on the jacket.

Delbanco Meyer Wigs: 1, 7, 14, 29, 30, 33.
Gay Girl Wigs: 2, 15.
Ginchywig Division of Clynol Ltd.: 32, 35.
Jantzen: 31.
Regina Creations: 27.
Robert Fielding Wigs: 17.
Steiner Organization: 6.
Wig Marla: 5, 18, 19, 34

Joanne Gale

Index